ASSUMPTIONS
CAN MISLEAD

ASSUMPTIONS CAN MISLEAD

*Failures in Health Care
and Elsewhere*

* * *

M. C. Dye

Order this book online at www.trafford.com
or email orders@trafford.com

Most Trafford titles are also available at major online book retailers.

Printed in the United States of America.

ISBN: 978-1-4669-8769-2 (sc)
ISBN: 978-1-4669-8770-8 (e)

Library of Congress Control Number: 2013905727

Trafford rev. 05/28/2013

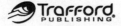 www.trafford.com

North America & international
toll-free: 1 888 232 4444 (USA & Canada)
fax: 812 355 4082

To the memory
of my Dad
W. J. Paul Dye, M.D., F.A.C.S.
a quintessential country doctor
who understood the art of listening

To the memory
of Ida Jean Orlando, R.N., M.A.
my teacher, mentor, and friend

To David Dunham
my husband and remarkable partner
without whose assistance
this book might not
have been possible

Author's Note

All stories in this book are true. If the story is referred to in the Notes and References, all information remains the same as noted there.

Except for Ida Orlando, myself, family, and friends, the names and identifying characteristics of all others are changed to protect their identity. The format separates specific stories from discussion. Memories in discussions are presented as accurately as possible.

Unless otherwise noted, all doctors referred to in this book are physicians.

Contents

Acknowledgments

This book would not have been written if I had not been a student, then a colleague and close friend of Ida Orlando (1926-2007), whose theory is the basis of this book. I believed her work needed to reach health care, including medical care, and it needed to reach the general public. It is impossible for me to adequately thank Ida Orlando for what she offered us through her theory. Those who read this book may also find themselves thanking her. She deserves the utmost praise.

At first Ida was not sure this book made sense. She believed the general public would have difficulty carrying out her theory "because," she said, "it takes discipline." I agreed that without thought it can be difficult. However, with further discussion she supported the book because she knew I planned to write about it through true stories, and she knew I was thoroughly familiar with her theory including the difficulties in carrying it out in practice. She eagerly awaited my first presentation of her theory to the general public in a Dinner Lecture Series at the Wellesley College Club on the college campus in 2008. Unfortunately she died before then. Her husband, Bob Pelletier, a few of her friends and nursing colleagues, some of my family, and people from the general public attended. She would have loved knowing that all responded very favorably. Many of them made a special effort to share their thoughts with me immediately after the lecture.

The lecture at Wellesley College would not have been possible had I not been asked by Andele Novak from the College Club to be one of the speakers in that Dinner Lecture Series. I am enormously grateful to Andele for that invitation which was my first opportunity to share Orlando's theory with the general public. Their response convinced me that Orlando's theory could be understood and even welcomed by those outside of health care. Their eager response bolstered me as I moved ahead, collected more stories, and began to write the first few chapters. That marvelous evening included a delicious dinner. Andele deserves immense credit for arranging an evening that went so smoothly and was so enjoyed by all.

Special thanks to Bob Pelletier for his continuing support. Though I did not need any more information about Ida's work, after the Wellesley lecture Bob offered to give me all of Ida's papers that were at their house. "Come on down and get them, they're yours." I declined but thanked him for his generosity. Through many phone calls he told me how enthusiastic he was about the book, and he shared many wonderful memories about Ida. Unfortunately, he also died before the book was completed.

For about a decade beginning in the mid-nineties I worked as a consultant in Orlando Theory with the Nursing Department at New Hampshire Hospital, an acute psychiatric hospital with a major affiliation with the Geisel School of Medicine at Dartmouth. The Nursing Department had decided to put Orlando Theory into practice. It became clear that Orlando Theory was easy to understand, but for various reasons, including issues involving assumptions, it was not easy to practice. I am grateful to the dedicated staff at New Hampshire Hospital who shared with me their struggles and successes in putting Orlando Theory into practice. From them I learned much more than I ever expected.

Because of my work with the New Hampshire Hospital staff, by the time I left the consulting position in 2006 I decided to delve more into the issues of assumptions as relevant to Orlando Theory by writing this book. By then I realized that the struggles in putting Orlando Theory into practice needed much more consideration, and that the theory was relevant for a wider audience: health care in general, medical care, and the general public. I told Ida Orlando about my plan a few weeks before she died in 2007. It was in the spring of the following year that I took her theory to the general public in my presentation at the Wellesley College Club.

Another supporter of this book was Florence Wald (1917-2008) who is credited with bringing the hospice movement to the United States from England. Over the years we had stayed in contact. She telephoned me shortly after a visit with Ida at her home in Massachusetts which led to a conversation about Ida and her theory. Florence was familiar with Orlando Theory. Ida, Florence, and I were at the Yale University School of Nursing during some of the same years. In a later telephone conversation with Florence I told her about my book. She understood that I valued her support which she offered during that conversation.

I enormously appreciate the enthusiasm and meticulous reviews from three critique readers, all experts in their fields: Karen

Baker, Clapham Murray, and Robert M. Vidaver, M.D. They were gracious to take time from their busy schedules. Other than my line editor and myself, these three critique readers were the first to read the book in its entirety. Their comments were invaluable, encouraging, and enriching. All recognized the importance of the content and how various themes played out through the stories. I also immensely appreciate that they wrote paragraphs in support of the book.

For nineteen years Karen Baker has owned the Country Bookseller, an independent book store. When the store's early popularity led Karen to realize she needed a larger store, many volunteers from the local and surrounding towns formed a human chain to pass each book a block and a half through the center of town from the former store to the new store. The process was slowed only by those who read the covers as the books passed through their hands. Karen Baker knows literature.

Clapham Murray is a veteran character actor whose performances my husband and I have enjoyed for many years at the Barnstormers Theater, America's oldest professional summer theater. He is Professor Emeritus of Theater Arts at New England College and its branch in Arundel, Sussex, England. He is the author of *The Making of Daniel*, an Amazon-Kindle book, and he was in the movie *In the Bedroom* produced a few years ago. Clapham Murray knows stories and story-telling.

Robert M. Vidaver, M.D., is Professor Emeritus of the Geisel School of Medicine at Dartmouth. From 1988 to 2008 he was Medical Director of New Hampshire Hospital, the acute psychiatric hospital affiliated with the Geisel School of Medicine, and Professor and Vice-Chair of the Department of Psychiatry. From 1988 to the present he has been serving as the Commissioner's Designee to the New Hampshire Board of Medicine. Dr. Robert M. Vidaver knows health care.

I have not included by name many family, friends, and colleagues who supported and encouraged me throughout my writing this book, only because the list is amazingly long and I do not want to miss anyone who may feel they should have been included. I can't count the number of times I'd go to town to get the mail and be stopped by one or more people whose comments included: how's the book coming; how far along are you now; I can't wait to read it; when will it be published; can I get a signed copy. I can't thank them enough.

When I first told David Dunham, my husband, that I was going to write a book about Orlando's theory through true stories, neither he nor I had any idea how essential he would become in the process from its inception to its publication. He knew about Ida and Bob through my telephone conversations with Ida during which she'd ask about David, and I'd ask about Bob. Through us they'd share their interests, such as how climate change seemed to be affecting birds in our yards. Both knew about Ida's theory, and both knew Ida and I had a commitment to having this book published.

I had met Bob a few times, had occasionally talked with him by phone, and he and Ida had once stopped to visit with me on their way north to a winter vacation. But the following warmed my heart as much as it took me by surprise. At the Wellesley College Club lecture I noticed Bob and his group coming through the outer door, so I went over to greet them as they entered the lobby. Bob looked at me and immediately said, "Hi, Mimi, where's David?" I motioned David over, and they stayed together throughout the evening. David's friendship was enormously supportive to Bob who was grieving Ida's loss which had occurred only four months prior to that evening.

When I began writing the first chapters soon after that lecture, David offered to be my line editor and to comment on anything I wrote. He had been praised as a line editor by others, we already worked well together on writing and other relevant matters, so I accepted his offer. He knew he would be helping me with my computer, because I invariably rely on him to sort out my computer struggles.

As time went on I realized that I had not only an in-house line editor and computer consultant, I had a partner who was available to me any time I needed his advice. No matter what time of day, or what he was doing, he took time to listen to my thoughts and ruminations, and he'd offer advice. He told a friend that we occasionally had "spirited discussions" about his editorial suggestions, but we both agreed that the final version should be mine. His involvement was not only emotionally supportive, his line editing kept the writing crisp, and our discussions helped to keep me focused. If he believed some content was not clear, I would rewrite it.

Then it came time to electronically send the manuscript to Trafford Publishing. That is way beyond my competence. David had already worked on the book cover with Maryann Evans at Kingswood Press, where he has for many years been a printer, so he and Maryann also agreed to work together to put the manuscript into the proper format to electronically send it to Trafford. I am grateful to Bill Swaffield, owner of Kingswood Press, for his invaluable assistance, and to Maryann and thank her for her expertise and commitment. Her involvement also made it possible to include my ideas before it reached Trafford.

I believe I would have found a way to write and publish this book by myself. But it would not have been the book that it is without David's various skills, his emotional support, and his commitment to the ultimate product. There are not enough words to thank him. That he is on the dedication page as well as what I said there is a measure of my thanks.

Preface

Assumptions are interwoven into the very fabric of our lives. When we make an assumption we take something for granted. We accept it as fact. Incorrect assumptions can have powerful effects on our emotions and our lives. Incorrect assumptions can lead us astray. If we fail to recognize our incorrect assumptions we may find ourselves in situations that range anywhere from minor misunderstandings to disastrous outcomes.

Medical errors are a serious problem in health care.[1] Misunderstandings anywhere in the health care system can lead to patient complications, even death. Our medical professionals need to be aware of incorrect assumptions that can compromise the process of making accurate diagnoses, reasonable treatment plans, and carrying out those plans.

This book includes innumerable stories about people of all ages in a wide variety of situations in health care and elsewhere. All the stories are true. Through these stories the book describes and discusses our need to be understood, the types of assumptions we make, and how Orlando Theory[2] can help us recognize assumptions before we act on them. This is a book about us and how our assumptions affect us.

This book also includes information on how our minds influence our health and our immune systems. By how we hear our doctors and how we understand ourselves, we sometimes make and act on incorrect assumptions about our health. We can even talk to our T-cells, a form of biofeedback, to help us deal with bacteria in infections, viruses, and cancer. T-cells are important fighters in the body's immune response to foreign cells.[3]

We need to have others who will listen and know what we mean. Incorrect assumptions can prevent accurate listening and reasonable responses. Orlando Theory offers us a way to listen and communicate clearly and accurately. It can remind us to be aware of our assumptions when we are in health care and elsewhere. Depending on the context, for ease in understanding, in this book Orlando Theory is also any of the following: the Orlando Communication Model, the Orlando Model, or the Model.

In recent years I presented Orlando Theory to a nursing school conference and to two conferences at New Hampshire Hospital, an acute psychiatric hospital affiliated with the Geisel School of Medicine at Dartmouth. Another presentation was in a Dinner Lecture Series at the Wellesley College Club on the Wellesley College campus. Lively discussions and various questions followed.

At one of the hospital conferences one participant seemed angry and demanded to know why schools of nursing, medicine, and business don't know about this. She well understood that using Orlando Theory can prevent serious errors in health care. Another participant said she was familiar with the content and, because she felt it was so valuable in her personal life, came to the conference to learn more. Three student teachers at the Wellesley College Club lecture said they were going to begin to use what they learned from the presentation in their student teaching the very next day.

Various students and colleagues in health care have encouraged me to write this book to respond to the many questions and to the need for clarification about Orlando Theory. They recognize its value in health care and elsewhere, but find it especially difficult to use in intensely emotional situations, the very situations where clear communication is not only needed, but may be essential to prevent violence or to save a life.

Ida Orlando and I had many conversations about the difficulty health care students had in learning her theory. Our discussions inevitably returned to the issue of assumptions. Because she believed it takes discipline to recognize when we are making or acting on an assumption, she supported my bringing this issue to the general public. She was well aware that any of us in our daily lives can too easily act on assumptions that may adversely affect us.

My professional and personal relationship with Ida Orlando, my life experiences and professional career in mental health (faculty, administrator, supervisor, clinician), and many years as a psychotherapist have made it possible for me to write this book.

ASSUMPTIONS
CAN MISLEAD

1. Orlando's Model

It was 8:03 a.m. I had just arrived at my office at a rural mental health service. The phone rang. Our secretary said, "Dr. McKay is at the hospital. He wants to talk with you. He says it's urgent." "Put him on," I said. He asked me to come to the hospital immediately because Mavis, my patient whom he admitted a couple nights ago, had pulled the fire alarm. "We need to get her out of here." I assured him I'd be right over. As I arrived I was surrounded by Dr. McKay and some nurses. Firemen were clumping around in their tall black boots, yellow slickers, and firemen's hats. A couple policemen watched me as I went over to Dr. McKay. He immediately told me that Mavis had pulled the fire alarm early this morning. He wanted me to transfer her to the state psychiatric hospital. I said I'd talk with her.

As I walked into her room I saw a small, slightly gray haired woman in her pale blue, rumpled gown, looking forlorn, sitting on the side of the bed. She quickly looked up, then said "Hi" as she smiled in recognition of me. I acknowledged her also with a smile, a nod and "Good morning." I sat down in the chair near the bed, asked her how she was, and how the night went. "I'm okay now." She briefly hesitated, then continued. "A while ago I woke up. It was dark. I didn't know where I was. I was scared. I got out of bed, went into the hall, but I still couldn't figure out where I was. I saw the fire alarm and pulled it." She looked thoughtful, then continued. "When I was a little girl, my mother told me if I ever got lost to find a policeman or a fireman, or even pull a fire alarm, and they would come and help me." "What happened then?" I asked. "A nurse came and brought me back to my room."

In further conversation Mavis said she knew she was in the local hospital. She knew its name. She knew she had been admitted for a change in medication because she had been hearing voices, and her thoughts had been confused. She admitted feeling anxious and distressed because the nurse didn't talk with her, only returned her to her room. She thought the nurse was angry with her. She had not seen anyone since then. She was no longer hearing voices, and her thoughts were no longer confused. She wanted to see her husband. She wanted to go home.

I reassured her I would talk with Dr. McKay, and we would have her husband come and take her home. We agreed it was indeed good news that the medication change was successful. She calmed down during our conversation. She was pleased that she would be discharged and would be going home. I was with her less than ten minutes.

Dr. McKay met me on my way down the hall. He urgently asked me when I could send her to the psychiatric hospital. I told him she no longer needed any hospital. I explained why she pulled the alarm and added that she was no longer confused or hearing voices. The medication change was working. Mavis knew who she was, where she was, why she had been admitted, and she knew that it was now morning. I said she could be discharged whenever her husband could come, and she was eager to go home. He acknowledged what I said, went and talked with her, then called her husband who came for her.

* * *

When Dr. McKay called me to come to the hospital, he had already made the assumption that the symptoms for which he had admitted Mavis had contributed to her pulling the fire alarm. Since the nurse who led her back to her room had not talked with her, it appears that she had made the same assumption.

When you make assumptions you take your thoughts and/or feelings to be a true version of the situation. You take them for granted without checking them out, without verifying them for accuracy.

Yale professor Ida Orlando discovered that successful communication is a process which includes five ingredients that flow from one to the other. The first is *Perceptions*, what we are aware of through our senses: what we see, hear, taste, touch, or smell. Being keenly aware of our perceptions is very important because this is the first information we receive. When we start interpreting what we have perceived, we are in the second and third ingredients, *Thoughts* and/or *Feelings*. The fourth ingredient is *Validation*, verifying accurate understanding of a situation. The fifth is *Action*, which should only be taken after verification. That action should also be verified to ascertain whether or not it has been relevant to the situation.

Had Dr. McKay transferred Mavis to the psychiatric hospital without including her version of the situation, he would have been acting on an inaccurate, unverified assumption. It took only a few brief questions for her to tell me why she pulled the alarm and give me the information that indicated she no longer needed any hospital and was capable of returning home.

* * *

Dr. Daley saw Gertrude, a middle-aged woman neatly dressed in dark brown slacks and a red sweater, looking at a book while waiting to see him. He was treating her for a chronic medical condition. He felt encouraged that her symptoms were not preventing her from reading.

They had developed a comfortable relationship. So, as she walked into his office, he asked her what she was reading. She hesitated, then volunteered that she could not read or write English. She admitted she often brought a book because she did not want to be drawn into conversations. She further admitted that for some time she had wanted to talk about this with him, but had felt too ashamed to bring it up.

He was puzzled. He knew she had come from Germany. Though she was not working, she had told him she had held executive positions here. So he asked how she had managed to do this. She said that her son, who can read and write English, handled all her paperwork. When she was at work, secretaries typed her dictations and filled out papers. She wanted to look for another job, but had been struggling with the ever present fear she'd be found out. She asked if he knew of any courses she could take to learn to read and write English. With the help of his staff she successfully attended such a program, and was accepted in a job that required writing skills. Dr. Daley and his staff were thrilled when Gertrude proudly read and filled out new office forms at an office visit a few months later. It had never occurred to them to question her when she had previously taken such forms home.

* * *

Dr. McKay and Mavis with the fire alarm, and Dr. Daley and Gertrude with her book, show how easy it is to make assumptions that can mislead. Neither Dr. McKay nor Dr. Daley ever considered that they were making incorrect assumptions. Action should only be taken after you validated that you have an accurate understanding about a situation. In these two stories the patients volunteered the needed information before actions were taken, Mavis with me, Gertrude with Dr. Daley.

* * *

Betsy Lehman, age thirty-nine, mother of two children, had worked at *The Boston Globe* newspaper for over a decade. She had covered topics ranging from research to relationship issues between health care professionals and their patients. When she learned she had advanced breast cancer she carefully studied her options. She chose to undergo an experimental treatment offered at the Dana-Farber Cancer Institute in Boston, Massachusetts, a prestigious cancer center associated with Harvard Medical School. Her treatment plan was a high dose of chemotherapy to be given over four days.

After the first day's treatment a nurse found her weepy, frightened, anxious, unable to keep down fluids, and intensely protesting the discharge plan to send her home. Betsy said she did not know what was wrong, but something was very wrong. She felt terrible and attempted to describe her symptoms. She did not feel ready to go home. She did not believe her caregivers were listening to her. She felt desperate. So she telephoned a friend who was a hospital social worker. Only the answering machine responded. She left the following message: "I'm feeling very frightened, very upset. I don't know what's wrong, but something's wrong." It was too late. Within the next hour she died. No one had responded to her frantic efforts to be heard.

Betsy Lehman had developed severe symptoms related to the chemotherapy. An investigation into her death revealed that she had been given a huge dose that should have been equally divided over four days. Her dose was four times the required dose. The pharmacy had failed to catch the error. Furthermore, her physicians did not respond to abnormal readings from a blood test, nor did they ask for interpretation of an electrocardiogram from a cardiologist, both of which would have supported Betsy's concerns that her situation was critical and needed an immediate response.

The investigation highlighted that Betsy's account of her symptoms were as important as any physical data. The investigation stated that the failure of caregivers to adequately respond to her perceptions and anxieties was a factor in her death. It appeared that at least five hospital staff failed to figure out that the therapy was killing her.[1]

* * *

It is well known that chemotherapy has side effects that can make people feel terrible. Yet here we have an intelligent journalist, knowledgeable about health care, who communicated as clearly and emphatically as she could about feeling worse than what might be expected. Her inability to hold down fluids, the abnormal blood tests, and the electrocardiogram supported her concerns. Even then no one listened and responded.

The Orlando Model emphasizes the importance of incorporating in treatment plans what the patient says, especially in a red flag situation such as this. It appeared that Betsy's caregivers relied on their knowledge and expectations about side effects of chemotherapy, rather than responding to Betsy's distress supported by the physical data. Assumptions can mislead. Failures occur in health care, sometimes with disastrous, tragic results.

* * *

The ringing phone pulled me from my book. It was 10:35 p.m. and I was on call. "This is the hospital. The sheriff is on his way from the jail. He's bringing an inmate he wants you to see in the emergency room. Can you come right in?" I closed my book. "Sure, I'll be there in 10 to 15 minutes."

The emergency room door swished opened as I walked through and scanned the scene in front of me. The charge nurse nodded and called over the sheriff. A prison guard was standing erect beside a door to one of the examining rooms. As the sheriff walked with me to meet the guard he said Kevin had trashed his cell. I started to open the door. The guard put up his hand and stopped me. "I'm going in with you." "No," I said. "I want to see him alone." The guard stared at me. "I don't think it's safe." "Well," I said, "you can watch through the door window. If anything happens, then you can come in." He hesitated, then nodded because I was already half way through the door and closing it on him.

Sitting in a chair just inside the door with his back to the wall was a tall guy in scruffy jeans and a black jacket. His dark hair was rumpled and he hadn't shaved for a day or so. His handcuffed hands were in his lap. His ankles were shackled with a short chain permitting only short steps. I immediately sat down in the chair beside him, my back also to the wall. Since we were to the left of the door facing the back of the room, the guard couldn't see either of us.

Kevin turned his head and stared at me. "I'm from the mental health service. I'm on call." He continued to look at me. "I'm your ally. I'm here to help you any way I can." I reached in my pocket, pulled out my professional card and held it toward him. Because both hands were held together by handcuffs he reached out and took the card in both hands. He slowly read it then turned and faced me again. "They told me you trashed your cell." Silence. "Is that really true?" Kevin nodded and with emphasis said "Yes." He put my card in his jacket pocket. "Why did you trash your cell?" He responded intensely with barely a pause. "I wanted to call my lawyer. I trashed my cell because they wouldn't let me call my lawyer." I was stunned and incredulous. "You have a right to call your lawyer. I'll see to it that they let you call your lawyer." He looked away, then back at me. "Is that the only reason you trashed your cell?" "Yes, it's the only reason." "Can you promise me you won't trash your cell again if they allow you to call your lawyer?" "Yes," he said with emphasis. I kept looking at him. "For sure you can make that promise?" "Yes, I can make that promise. If they let me call my lawyer I won't trash my cell again." His voice had softened but remained firm.

Then I asked various questions explaining that I otherwise needed to know how he was. He answered easily. No hallucinations. No delusions. He knew the approximate time, where he was and who he was. "I'll tell them you have every right to call your lawyer and they have to let you do that. Is there anything else you want to say or ask me before I go?" "No," he said with a softer tone. "Take care of yourself." He acknowledged my departing words with a nod.

The sheriff and guard looked at me as soon as I opened the door. "He promises he won't trash his cell again if you let him call his lawyer. I believe him. He has a legal right to call his lawyer, so let him do that." They both looked down at me then at each other. The sheriff responded. "We'll let him do that." I nodded, "Good. Thanks." Then I signed off with the emergency room staff and left.

At the mental health service a couple days later my office phone rang. "There's a man here who wants to see you, but he won't give his name or say what he wants." Within a few minutes I rounded the corner into the waiting room. There he was. His hair was combed. He had shaved, and he looked sharp in his clean dungarees and dark green sweater. Kevin got up as I reached him and asked how he was. "I'm good, I'm good," he said with a grin. "You want an appointment?" "No, I don't want an appointment. I just came over to thank you." "They let you call your lawyer?" "Yes, and I got out the next day." "Well, good. Is there anything else I can do for you?" "No, I really just came over to see you and thank you." I nodded. "I appreciate that. Now that you know where we are, do let us know if I or any of us can be of help to you." We shook hands as he quietly left with a nod and a wave.

* * *

Mavis' behavior was logical and reasonable, but no one asked her why she pulled the fire alarm. They assumed she was out of control. "Call mental health!" She told me she believed the nurse was angry with her. Her doctor hadn't even come to see her. She wanted to go home. She wanted to get out of there. It is not unusual to hear people say they are more upset with their health care than they may be about the symptoms that brought them to that care.

Gertrude felt ashamed to admit she couldn't read or write English. She and others who feel ashamed are often reluctant to mention issues that need to be addressed.

Kevin's request to call his lawyer was not only reasonable. It is his legal right. When his request was not granted he became furious and trashed his cell. "He's out of control! Take him to the emergency room! Call mental health!" More people became involved: the sheriff, another guard, the emergency room staff, and mental health.

Betsy Lehman attempted to describe her symptoms and emphasize her worry and concerns. Her physical data supported her situation as being very serious. Her situation escalated as did those of Mavis and Kevin. But when no one really understood and pursued the critical nature of Betsy's symptoms, she died.

When professionals and others behave from inaccurate, unverified assumptions situations can escalate. More time and people may become involved. All kinds of emotions are triggered.

Even then the crucial data can be overlooked. For Betsy Lehman it was too late.

2. Tell Me Your Story

There are good listeners in health care and elsewhere. My grandfathers and my father were physicians before modern technology was available. They had to listen carefully to their patients. When combined with physical exams, they knew their patients' stories offered essential information from which to make accurate diagnoses and treatment plans. They also knew their patients needed to be comfortable enough to talk openly with them. Remember Gertrude with Dr. Daley? She had not told him she could not read or write English until she became comfortable with him, and he gave her an opening by asking her what she was reading.

Pop Clow, my maternal grandfather, lived less than a mile from us. Some of my earliest memories of him are when I was about five and I would visit him in his office in his house. Not wanting to startle him I would quietly tiptoe down the hall into his office. He would look up from his desk, beckon me to come in, then lift me up onto his knees. He would look at me with a mischievous grin and in his booming voice say: "Well now Molly, how are things going for you? What stories do you have for me today?" Then he'd listen, ask questions and listen some more. This was special not just because he called me Molly and wouldn't let anyone else do so, but because he'd take the time to listen and understand. Years later, when I returned as a mental health professional, some of his former patients told me they revered him because he cared about them through his listening, his empathy, and his diagnostic and therapeutic skills.

My Dad also knew the importance of listening to his patients. I accompanied him on many house calls. Though not included in the medical part of the visit, I was with him when patients would continue to talk with him on his way in and out of their houses. As with my grandfather, they appreciated his surgical and medical skills, but also, as they told me later, they appreciated his taking the time to listen and understand what they were trying to say. They knew what they said offered crucial information he needed in order to make correct diagnoses and treatment plans. They also knew he cared about them by the way he listened.

I understood this because from the time I was a little kid he always listened well to me. If needed, he would patiently ask then listen to be sure he was clear about what I was trying to say. He died when I was a teenager. His loss was huge. It took years for me to truly realize the power of careful listening which I first learned from him.

Some folks are just naturally good listeners. Even then it can take considerable effort to understand what some people are trying to say. Encouraging them to tell their stories as completely as possible may sometimes be the only way to understand what they wish to convey.

* * *

Dr. Dobkin went to the waiting room. He called out the name of his next patient. A tall man in a worn sport coat got up. "Do you remember me?" he said as he followed Dr Dobkin into the examining room. "You saw me a couple of times when I had the stroke. Maybe four years ago." Dr. Dobkin asked Earl to refresh his memory and told his secretary to get Earl's old hospital chart.

As soon as they entered the examining room Earl pushed his chair against the door blocking passage. "All you guys start waving goodbye before I'm finished. Now that I've got you, I want some answers." Dr. Dobkin sat back in his chair to show he was ready to listen. "Tell me how I can help you."

"It's this left side that's numb all the time . . . it's been doing it since the stroke . . . I want to know what this numbness is about." Earl looked at Dobkin as if he were challenging him. Dr. Dobkin asked numerous questions to sort through information about the numbness. It felt like pins and needles. It fluctuated, but was not painful. "It's numb and I want to know what it is," Earl emphasized.

The secretary knocked on the door but was unable to open it. Earl pulled his chair aside and let in the secretary with the old chart. As soon as she left he pushed his chair back against the door. He stayed silent while Dr. Dobkin reviewed the chart. Now he remembered him. Earl had been hospitalized for a stroke. He had been a reluctant patient. Despite symptoms from the stroke such as slamming his left shoulder or hip when walking through a door frame he denied anything was wrong. Each morning he had insisted he could go home. Most of his symptoms cleared within a week. An abnormal heart rhythm had resulted in the upper left heart chamber filling with tiny blood clots. One had traveled to his brain and caused his stroke.

Dr. Dobkin carefully explained how his stroke could lead to the tingling sensations he was feeling. Earl listened attentively, but Dobkin noted nothing had changed in Earl's demeanor. He continued by adding that one of several medications might reduce the numbness but they could have side effects that could impair his memory or cause impotence. Might that be worse than the tingling? Earl agreed. "So the tingling bothers you, but not so much that you can't live with it," Dobkins said mostly to himself. "Been living with it, but I don't want it," Earl replied.

After all this and nothing had changed. Dr. Dobkin began to wonder if maybe this stout, bullheaded man was scared. "Are you worried about the numbness because it reminds you of your stroke?" Earl quietly answered, "Yes." Dr. Dobkin continued, "Do you think that the tingling is a sign that you're going to have another stroke?" Earl lowered his head and softly responded with watery eyes, "Yes." He added that for the previous three and a half years he believed he was living with a time bomb.

Dr. Dobkin handed him some tissues. "Let me make sure you understand this." Then he went on to explain how the atrial fibrillation allowed a clot to form that had reached a small artery in his head and caused the stroke. However, his heartbeat since the stroke was regular because Earl had been responsibly taking the prescribed heart medication. As long as he kept taking the medication, the tingling and numbness were only a reminder of the past, nothing more. "It doesn't mean I'll have another stroke? You're telling me I won't have another stroke?" Dobkins told him his risk for another stroke was no more than anyone his age. Earl slammed his hand down on the arm of the chair. "Now you've got it!" He stood, pulled aside the chair, opened the door and strutted out of the office, finally satisfied with the visit.

Dr. Dobkin knew the importance of ascertaining the real reason for Earl's concern. He made no unverified assumptions. He doggedly stayed with Earl until he knew by Earl's verbal and nonverbal behavior that he had ascertained and met Earl's need. As professor of clinical neurology, Dr. Dobkin had examined neurology candidates the previous week. He failed three out of seven who had not asked enough questions to understand what their patients meant by their complaints. The flunked physicians had turned to medical technology with high cost and risk instead of taking more time with their patients to tease out the meaning of their complaints.[1]

* * *

Making the effort to understand and adequately respond to someone's need can sometimes save time, expense, and the involvement of other people. Dr. Dobkin finally understood and resolved Earl's concern. Earl was not likely to return for the same reason. Because the staff at the jail did not respond to Kevin's clearly stated reasonable request to call his lawyer, more time, expense and people were involved.

* * *

Deborah Smith was a nurse who periodically flew across the country to attend classes in California. On one of the flights the loud speaker asked for any medical personnel to please identify themselves to any of the cabin crew. Deborah responded. She learned that a man wearing a gray hooded sweatshirt with the hood over his head had boarded the plane with his head down and that he had not acknowledged any of the crew who had spoken to him. After takeoff he had gone to the back lavatory and locked himself in. Three hours later he was still there and the crew wanted to know if he was all right. The line was backing up for the front lavatory by frustrated passengers who didn't understand why the back lavatory was locked.

The flight attendant looked panicked. Deborah felt anxious and began to consider the worst case scenario. Had he tried to commit suicide? Was he psychotic? Had he smuggled in a firearm? No, security would have found any weapons.

Deborah had the flight attendant knock on the door and ask him to name any medications he was taking. He answered that he was on a medication, but neither Deborah nor a doctor there knew the medication. So the flight attendant told him a nurse wanted to talk with him. Debbie knocked on the door. "Hello, my name is Debbie. I'm a nurse. I want to help you if I can. What is your name?" "Arthur," was the response. "I really want to try and help you, but it's very difficult to talk through the door with the plane engines. Could you come out, and we can sit down and talk? Look, I'll talk to you all the way to Los Angeles if you want."

"I don't know. Maybe in five to ten minutes." Five minutes passed. Debbie knocked on the door and announced herself again. She asked if they could talk "out here in the plane." Arthur replied that there would be no place to sit. Debbie assured him that the cabin crew had cleared the entire last row so they could sit and talk privately. "If I come out everyone out there will be looking at me and wondering what was going on and what was wrong with me."

"Arthur," said Debbie, "most of the people out here are just wanting to use the bathroom. Everybody else is facing the other way, and they don't care what you are doing." Debbie ordered the people lined up for the lavatory to step aside. Gradually the lock slid off and the door slowly opened. The hood on his gray sweatshirt was still pulled over his head. He towered over Debbie. She identified herself and extended her hand to indicate the last row of seats. Arthur quietly came out of the lavatory and sat in the aisle seat.

Debbie knelt down next to him, asked how he was and what could she do to help him. He said he had an upset stomach. He denied the offer of ginger ale or any other drink. He just wanted to lie down across the three seats and sleep. Debbie assured him that was fine and to tell any of the crew to call her if he needed her again. He nodded, curled up in the seats and soon fell asleep. He slept all the way through landing with no further issues for Debbie or the crew.[2]

* * *

The Orlando Model tells us we cannot assume we have adequately responded to someone's need until we can verify that our actions have adequately responded to the need. Verification includes the person's behavior changing for the better and, if possible, verbal acknowledgment that our actions did respond to the need. Earl verbally acknowledged what Dr. Dobkin said about his stroke, and he looked enormously relieved. Arthur's coming out of the lavatory and sleeping during the rest of the plane flight was verification enough that Debbie had adequately responded to his need.

3. Orlando's Enigma

So who was Ida Orlando and how did she discover this communication model? Already a nurse with previous work experience, Ida was about ready to graduate from Teacher's College, Columbia University with a masters degree in mental health consultation. The Director of the Psychiatric Mental Health Program at the Yale University School of Nursing, another graduate program, asked the Director at Columbia whom she might hire to come to Yale to integrate mental health concepts in nursing. She was told to hire Ida Orlando, and if Ida accepted, she'd be lucky to get her.

Ida accepted. And so, in 1954, the Yale School of Nursing was awarded a five year grant by the National Institute of Mental Health (N.I.M.H.) for Ida Orlando to integrate mental health concepts into a basic nursing curriculum. The curriculum was Yale's three year Master of Nursing (M.N.) Program. The students in this program were college graduates who had never been in nursing.

Ida was bright, energetic, and passionate about quality patient care. She knew most nursing successfully responded to patient needs. She also knew some patients were still in distress after their nursing care. She wanted to know why. She decided to go to the data itself.

She went to patient units all over the hospital, observed, and recorded nurse-patient interactions, putting each one on a card. Over at the School, the psychologists and psychiatrists told her she should take various mental health concepts and teach them to the students. She listened, nodded, and ignored their advice. She kept returning to the hospital and continued to meticulously observe and record nurse-patient interactions.

After she had about 2000 records of observations, she put them in one pile. She asked anyone who came by, faculty, students, nurses, to sort them into two piles, good nursing where patients' needs were met, and bad nursing where patients' needs were not met. No matter who sorted the pile, the good nursing pile was always the same, the bad nursing pile was always the same. Then she struggled to figure out why these piles were different.

At first she felt immersed in an impossible enigma. Both piles included the same nurses. Some included good listeners who successfully responded to their patients' needs most of the time. Their interactions were more often in the good nursing pile. Other nurses were less often successful and had more interactions in the bad nursing pile. Orlando believed that if she could discover what was inherent in the successful interactions, then she could teach such information to nurses. This would raise the overall quality of nursing care. Also, in being more consistently successful in responding to their patients' needs, nurses would be more satisfied with their work.

I was a student in that M.N. Program from 1955 to 1958. My classmates and I became Ida's students in this project as she sorted through the data from her initial observations and data from her and our nursing experiences. I share with you two classic stories from that era.

* * *

I was 5'2", average weight, with brown eyes and short, dark brown hair. Shirley, my classmate, was about 5'10", thin with bright blue eyes and long, shiny, light brown hair that hung softly over her shoulders. We were assigned to the same medical unit. We had the weekends off.

Late one Monday morning Ida returned to the conference room where we met with her to sort through our experiences. She wanted to know who had worked with Melvin, the elderly white-haired man in the corner room down the hall. He was now raising a ruckus with the nurses. He kept stating that he only wanted to have the nurse who had been with him last week. The nurses found him difficult over the weekend, and now he was demanding to have that nurse with the black tie that he had last week.

Black ties were part of our student uniform. It had to be one of us. I said Melvin was my patient Thursday and Friday, but not the beginning of the week. I had not been involved with him until I was assigned to him on Thursday. Shirley said he was her patient Monday through Wednesday, but she had been so busy with other patients Thursday and Friday, she hadn't seen him since Wednesday. Ida was puzzled, so she left to go talk with him. She was laughing when she returned to the conference room. He insisted he had only one nurse the whole week who was helpful to him, and he accurately described our student uniform. She asked him if possibly he had been mistaken and that he was talking about two different nurses. "Oh, no," he emphasized, "I had one nurse, the same nurse all week. She was great. She was helpful to me. If she is around, I want her again."

* * *

Because we had consistently responded to his needs, Melvin thought we were the same person. He didn't feel the nurses in the white uniforms were as helpful. He only wanted his nurse with the black tie.

By then Ida had discovered the ingredients in successful communication: *Perceptions* (raw data such as what we see or hear) lead us to our *Thoughts* and/or *Feelings*; *Validation* by the patient of the accuracy of our thoughts; then *Action* with further verification to ascertain whether or not we adequately responded to that patient's need. We had begun to be fairly consistent in successfully responding to our patients' needs. Melvin validated the success of our interactions with him with his comments to Ida.

* * *

On the Maternity Unit the nurse saw Amy grimacing as she looked into her room. Amy had delivered her baby by cesarean section. It was expected that she'd have pain from the stitches. So the nurse asked her if she were in pain. Amy nodded. Medication for pain had been prescribed. So the nurse left, returned with the medication, and put it on Amy's bedside table next to her glass of water. Amy was sitting up in bed, so the nurse told her to take it, then turned and walked out the door.

Sarah, one of my classmates, looked in, thought Amy didn't look well, and noticed the medication. She went in and asked Amy about it. Amy said it was for pain. Sarah asked why she had not taken it. Amy kept hesitating, obviously not wanting to answer. Ida always emphasized we must find out what the patient is thinking. So Sarah kept pressing.

Finally Amy blurted out that she had put on a girdle to look slimmer for her husband's visit. She was wearing the required binder that was used in those days, but Amy didn't feel the binder made her look as slim as she wanted. So she had put the girdle on over the binder. With some embarrassment she finally told Sarah that she had terrible pain after putting on the girdle. She believed she had torn the stitches.

"Let's take a look." Amy groaned as Sarah helped her slowly wriggle out of the girdle. Sarah undid the binder. The stitches were intact. The pressure was relieved. The pain disappeared. Sarah put the binder back on and Amy was more than willing to leave off the girdle. Amy sighed and said she felt so relieved. The nurse came by, saw the medication, and asked Amy why she had not taken it. Amy replied that she didn't have pain anymore. The nurse never asked why, just took the medication and left.

* * *

In this story Amy's nurse and physician expected Amy would need medication for pain. Amy acknowledged she was in pain, but felt unable to offer further information. The nurse assumed Amy's pain was from her operation and stitches and returned with the medication, assuming Amy would take it and that would solve the problem. The nurse was acting on unverified assumptions.

After working for a year after graduation, I returned to the Yale School of Nursing to work more with Ida, this time as a student in the two year Master of Science in Nursing (M.S.N.) psychiatric-mental health specialization. It seemed more challenging to work with psychiatric patients, especially when they were struggling with unbridled emotions and/or voices in their heads. We found that such patients responded well to us when we tried to ascertain what they needed from us. However, some of their situations were so intense, it was not possible to get verbal validation. As with Arthur who was talked out of the airplane lavatory and slept during the rest of the trip, non-verbal validation can sometimes suffice.

This next story took place at a psychiatric hospital where I was a consultant later in my career.

* * *

I was on one of the patient units. Phil, a mental health worker, recognized me and nodded. He had been in a staff session on another unit where I had presented the Orlando Model. Joe, a scruffy patient more than six feet tall, unkempt in dark rumpled clothes, unshaven for maybe a couple of days, came over. He looked down at me and in a gruff voice said, "Hi, I don't remember you." "Hi," I said. "I'm a nurse visiting the unit. How are things going for you?" "Good," he answered. "Are the staff helping you with what you need?" I asked. "Yes," he said.

Then he started telling me about an aunt of his whom he liked. He went into great detail about her and his relationship with her, including some of what they had done together. He was talking somewhat quickly and intensely. He was very involved in his story. As he was talking a female patient rushed by, pushing both of us aside. She said nothing. Her head was down, and she seemed preoccupied. She squeezed into a small space at the front of a counter just beyond me. She grabbed a pen and furiously began writing in what appeared to be a sign-out book. Then she quickly rushed off in another direction.

She startled me when she pushed me. I briefly glanced at her, then looked back at Joe. When she pushed Joe his voice became louder and more intense as he related his story about his aunt. He kept looking at me as he continued his story. Phil yelled over to Joe that he would soon be going to an appointment with the dermatologist. Joe's voice became even louder and more intense. He kept looking at me and went on with his story.

All of a sudden Phil and three other staff quickly came over and looked as if they were going to take over. I felt they were reacting to Joe's loud voice. Joe was still looking at me and with his intense, now louder voice, was continuing his story. Phil said, "Joe, you need to go to the dermatologist." I looked at Phil, put my hands up toward Phil and the other staff and said, "Let him finish his story." I looked again at Joe and said, "Finish your story, then you can go to the dermatologist." Joe said a few more sentences, not quite as loudly as before, and seemed to be finished. Then I said, "Now you can go to your appointment with the dermatologist. I've enjoyed talking with you."

I turned to Phil. "You're taking him to the dermatologist?" He nodded. Then he and Joe walked around the counter, on down the hall toward the door. Just before they reached the end of the hall, Joe turned around, smiled, waved at me and yelled, "You remind me of my mother." I smiled, nodded, and waved at him. He turned, and he and Phil continued out the door.

Within five minutes a new charge nurse came on for the evening shift. She knew who I was. She was able to arrange some time with me. So I told her about this incident with Joe, Phil, and the other staff who had come over with Phil in what looked like an attempt to protect me. She nodded and said, "Joe hit a staff member last night." She also told me that he does like his mother. She understood that I felt Joe had been reacting to being pushed and interrupted by the other patient, as well as having his story interrupted, yet again, by Phil.

* * *

Validation in this story was Joe's lowering his voice each time I did not let the interruptions take me away from listening to him. I made it clear that I wanted to hear the rest of his story. His comment to me about his mother, and the nurse saying he likes his mother, was further validation that I was adequately responding to his need to be heard and understood.

This story shows another point about the Orlando Model. It's important to stay focused, stay in the moment, and flow with what is happening. The Orlando Model does not expect us to think about each ingredient by name when we are in situations. But it does expect us to validate in some reasonable form that we are listening and understanding what this other person means and what this person wants from us.

Some time later I included this story about Joe and Phil in a conference about the Orlando Model. One of the participants wanted to know why I didn't ask Joe about his reaction to being pushed by the woman on her way to the counter. Had I done this I would not have been staying with what was most important to him, namely that I listen to his story. This is verified by his behavior. It would have been another distraction if I had interrupted his story to ask how he felt about being pushed by the lady leaving the counter. With his struggles keeping focus on his thoughts about the story he was telling, it is highly possible that he didn't even remember being pushed.

Joe consistently lowered his voice and settled down every time I refocused on listening to his story when either of us was distracted. Therefore it was obvious to me that he did not want to be interrupted in telling his story, or have me interrupted in listening to it. His intense, louder voice in response to each interruption, and lowering his voice each time he realized I was staying with him was evidence enough.

It is important to remember that Orlando emphasized that the person in the situation needs to stay in the moment and follow what occurs. The person involved in the situation is the only one who can fully comprehend what is occurring. When we worked with her as students, she continually emphasized that we needed to capture our thoughts and feelings which can only be done when one stays in the moment and in the flow of any interaction, most especially in an intense situation such as this. She would shake her head and correct anyone who called this the Orlando Process. "It's not the Orlando Process. It's not my process, it's their process! It's not what I think in the situation, it's what they think in the situation!" Therefore she insisted that analyzing situations should focus on what that person thought and felt in the situation, not what others think they might have said in the situation.

4. Urgent!

Because urgent situations involve people with desperate needs, urgent situations deserve, and sometimes demand, urgent responses. Some of the previous stories have involved situations with various degrees of urgency. But not all the participants in each situation have viewed their situation in the same way. As such, they have not considered the same solutions.

Dr. McKay wanted Mavis immediately transferred to a psychiatric hospital because she pulled the fire alarm. But Mavis only needed someone to tell her where she was. The guards at the jail swiftly brought Kevin to the hospital emergency service for a mental health evaluation. But he was furious only because they denied his reasonable request to telephone his lawyer. The medical professionals involved with Betsy Lehman and her chemotherapy not only failed to respond to her extreme psychological distress, they failed to correlate her distress and severe physical symptoms with the results of her blood test and the abnormal readings from her electrocardiogram. Betsy was so desperate to be understood that she telephoned a friend whom she hoped would come help her.

Even when people are in distress, if they are able to communicate, the Orlando Model expects us to talk with and listen to them, then verify that we understand what they are trying to say. Any actions then taken need verification in order to know if they have reasonably contributed to resolving those situations.

The next stories are presented to further address what happens when there is or is not an attempt to verify assumptions in urgent situations.

* * *

The birth of Edna's first child was extraordinarily painful. During the severe labor pains she had felt she couldn't breathe, and she had felt terrible pressure as if a cinder block had been put on her abdomen. She remembered the nurse trying to get her cooperation in moving down the delivery table. But she couldn't help the nurse. She felt scared and helpless. She had thought she would die.

She and her husband wanted more children. But she feared going through another similar experience. Then she heard about a conference to help women handle labor and delivery fears. She enrolled. There were twenty participants. She had heard the group would be small because the plan was for each of them to go through a simulated labor and delivery. One at a time they would lie on a mat, tightly wrap themselves in a blanket to simulate the feeling of abdominal pressure, then they would take slow, deep breaths which were designed to help them handle the labor pains.

Ten participants had been through the experience that morning. Edna was scheduled after lunch. At lunch she and the others shared their doubts about its helpfulness in getting through an actual birth. Even so, that afternoon Edna did as she was told. She lay down on the designated mat. It was hard, but warm from the previous person. She wrapped herself in the blanket that was given to her. Others were told to wrap her more tightly, which they did. Keri, the leader, offered encouragement with the breathing. "Slowly now, take one deep breath, slowly let it out, then repeat with more slow, deep breaths, one after another."

The room was quiet. "I can't breathe," Edna said to no one in particular. Keri responded, "Good, that's what a birthing experience feels like. Take another breath." Edna tried, but it looked as if she were trying to catch her breath. Others noticed that the blanket was very tight and they thought Edna was trying to wriggle. "I can't breathe!" "Exactly. That's the way it's supposed to be," emphasized Keri, "You will find your way through it."

This scenario continued for many more minutes. Edna turned pale. Her breaths became shallow, then stopped. Some thought she was holding her breath. She was not. By the time they unwrapped her and tried to revive her it was too late. Another needless death.

* * *

As with Betsy Lehman, Edna's words were not believed, not understood as a desperate cry indicating an emergency which needed careful thought as well as immediate attention.

* * *

Harold ran through the main door of the psychiatric hospital. The security guards turned as he yelled. "I'm going to kill someone if I don't get help!" Dan, a senior staff member ever alert to a raised voice, was in the lobby near the door. He turned and looked directly at Harold. "I heard you. I'll help you. Come. We can go into this room." Dan waved Harold to follow him. Since the security guards knew Dan they remained attentive, and did not follow.

As soon as Dan and Harold entered the room Dan spoke again. "What's the matter?" A long story bumbled forth. Harold said he and his wife could not stop arguing. Dan carefully listened. Harold's voice slowly softened as Dan continued to verify with various questions and statements that he understood Harold's concerns. "Where's your wife now?" Harold said he left her in the car. "Will you go get her so we can include her?" "OK, sure, I'll get her." They returned and Harold was willing to let her speak for herself. Finally the issues were sorted out enough for Harold and his wife to feel they could return home. Before they left, Dan asked Harold one final question. "Were you really going to kill someone?" "No, no, I felt like it. I wouldn't do that. I felt I was going to blow. I just needed some help."

* * *

Dan knows the Orlando Model. He is also thoughtful and brings an air of calm to urgent situations. He was alert to Harold's words, understood that Harold sought immediate help, and quickly indicated he would listen to him in another room where they would be away from others. Dan made no assumptions. He patiently listened, asked questions as needed to be sure he understood, then found an appropriate time to see if Harold were willing to include his wife. Since Harold was upset about that relationship, it was important to include her, but only when Harold felt able to do so. Dan respected Harold's thoughts and feelings throughout and verified that he understood him before suggesting any action. He did not let them leave until both felt they had sorted out enough issues to feel they were ready to go home.

The essence of the Orlando Model is as follows. Begin by being aware of your perceptions, information you receive through your senses. In this case it was what Dan saw and heard. Never assume. Stay in the moment. Flow with the situation. Follow that person's thoughts and feelings. With questions and statements continually verify as needed to be sure you fully understand before suggesting and/or taking any action. Share your thoughts and/or feelings as they are relevant to clarifying or resolving the situation. Include the person throughout. In some of the previous stories this was not done. Dan clearly focused on understanding what Harold was going through. He included him and ultimately his wife in sorting through and resolving their situation. He did not have them leave until both felt able to do so.

* * *

In April 2007 breaking news flooded the media about an acute situation at Virginia Tech in Blacksburg, Virginia. A lone gunman, referred to as the shooter, killed two students in one of the university dormitories. He evaded detection for over two hours, then killed another thirty people in another part of the campus before killing himself. Students were told in an e-mail to take precautions. But this e-mail was sent over two hours after the first shooting. It reached them at about the same time as the shooter entering Norris Hall where the mass killing occurred. Those on campus were warned too late. School officials had delayed the message because they believed the dormitory shooting was an isolated incident.

The police believed the first shooting was the result of a domestic dispute. Emily was one of the first two students killed. Shortly thereafter the police interviewed Heather, Emily's friend. She mentioned that Emily's boyfriend owned guns, and that he had recently taken her and Emily to the shooting range. Heather realized this information was being seized upon as supporting a domestic situation. She emphasized that Emily and her boyfriend had an amazing relationship, that he was not violent.

Despite that information, the police pursued Emily's boyfriend as the prime suspect. Because he was no longer there and they thought he was trying to leave the state, they immediately left the campus to try to find him.[1]

* * *

That all the Virginia Tech students were not told to take precautions until over two hours later tells us that the police did not appear to be considering any other possibilities that warranted a campus-wide alert. Surely if they had considered that a shooter might still be there, they would have remained and immediately warned all the people on campus about possible danger. Such a decision might have saved some lives. In focusing on Emily's boyfriend, the police acted on an unverified, incorrect assumption, which, once again, led to tragic results.

* * *

Two dispatchers from the California Highway Patrol received 911 calls reporting a fire on the south rim of Lake Tahoe. The first call was from a man who stated that he was on the Lake Tahoe Country Club golf course. He and others could see smoke coming off the mountain west of them. One of the dispatchers acknowledged the call. "Yeah. Yeah . . . they're doing a control burn there." "Thank you. Sorry to bother you," the caller quickly replied. Other calls were similar.

The smoke was not from a control burn. It was from a wildfire that ultimately destroyed 254 homes, some pets, and burned 3,100 acres of mountain wilderness. One of the men who lost his house said he was disgusted because "we knew this basin was a tinderbox." The fire started after an illegal campfire was built about a quarter mile south of Seneca Pond, a popular recreation area south of Lake Tahoe. It was eight more days before firefighters could contain the blaze. The cost of suppressing the fire was $12.1 million.

The Highway Patrol policy instructs dispatchers to keep callers on the line and transfer them to a local fire department in such situations. Because the dispatchers did not follow this policy, there was a crucial delay in responding to the fire. Commander Captain Gary Ross acknowledged that the dispatchers' dismissals of the initial reports caused a critically delayed response to the fire.[2]

* * *

Can previous training make a difference in how we respond? Training offers core information, but cannot include all possible variations that may occur, even in life and death situations. An emergency is not always recognized as an emergency. We saw this with Betsy Lehman who died from her chemotherapy, with Edna who died in her simulated birth experience, and with the dispatchers at Lake Tahoe. The police involved in the Virginia Tech situation understood there was an emergency, but they locked into their belief that Emily's boyfriend was the shooter. They did not expand their thinking to consider that another person might be the shooter and might still be on campus. It appears that these respondents never even considered that they might be acting on unverified, incorrect assumptions.

Dan recognized his situation as an emergency. He knew he needed to understand what was contributing to the emergency and what would resolve it. He knew the Orlando Model, so he made no assumptions. He continued to listen and ask questions, as needed, to clarify and verify the essence of the problem with Harold. Then he and Harold together worked on an immediate solution, namely to include Harold's wife in the discussion. The problematic issues were sorted out enough for Harold to calm down and for him and his wife to return home.

5. Tenacious Assumptions, Dogged Beliefs

Incorrect, unverified assumptions tend to be automatic and often tenacious. These next stories highlight types of situations where tenacious assumptions can be dogged beliefs.

* * *

Uncle Jacob had been a bachelor with no children. Aaron and Isaac were Jacob's only nephews. They hadn't seen each other much over the years, but they shared time together when they both attended Dartmouth College, and later with their families most summers at Uncle Jacob's estate in Maine. When Uncle Jacob died their lives became more intertwined. With a trust company they became successor co-trustees of the Jacob Zackner Trust. As co-executors they became involved with a law firm to handle legal matters. After certain monies were distributed to various designated recipients, Aaron and Isaac were to decide how to distribute the real estate and personal property. Since they were equal heirs, this would take careful consideration.

Successful in real estate, Uncle Jacob had acquired two large houses on expensive ocean front properties on the Maine coast. Though the houses were about a mile apart, the properties were contiguous. When both families were at the estate, they occasionally got together for various activities. But there were more than just these properties to consider.

A few years before his death, Uncle Jacob had become more and more concerned about the shoreline being less available to local fishermen, since so much of that land had been bought by wealthy families. He knew some of the fishermen who were struggling to find, or stay, on affordable shoreline from which to launch their fishing activities. To help them he bought some undeveloped shore property and an undeveloped island for them to use. He continually resisted pressure to rent either of these properties to people other than the local fishermen for whom he charged minimal rent.

Within the first few months of Uncle Jacob's death, assessors documented the value of all personal property and real estate. As co-executors Aaron and Isaac were continually requested to obtain various documents for their lawyer which he needed to complete the work for taxes and other obligations. Both nephews had been receiving the same letters. Isaac supported having Aaron respond to the requests because Aaron owned a logging business in northern Maine near his home, and he could find the time to get to Uncle Jacob's estate and bank where many of the documents were located. Aaron and their lawyer also kept in communication by phone. Isaac lived in Connecticut and was rarely available. He was frequently in Europe on business for the conglomerate for which he worked. As best as possible Aaron kept Isaac informed about the relevant issues.

It was summer now, and both were at the estate with their families. They belonged to a private country club, ate dinner, and often played bridge with their wives and others at the club in a social group they had been with for years. On this particular evening they were planning to meet their wives at the club for dinner and bridge. Because of different previous commitments, the men were coming in their own cars. Their wives would arrive together after a shopping afternoon farther down the coast. Aaron had just reviewed the law firm's letters and realized that in one letter their lawyer said, as equal heirs, he and Isaac should get together that summer to sort out the real estate and personal property. Their lawyer especially noted that they needed to make a decision about the shore and island properties the fishermen were using.

Aaron knew Uncle Jacob had talked with his own lawyer about plans to put those properties into conservation easements with the stipulation that they would only be used by the local fishermen who were in a co-op that could accept the properties as a gift. If the fishermen ultimately no longer intended to use either of these properties, then the following was to occur. The island would be given to a Maine island trust that protected such islands from development. The shore property would be forever protected from development by the conservation easement. Aaron knew that Uncle Jacob had not been able to finalize these plans before he died. He believed Uncle Jacob's wishes should be honored. Since Isaac had been away much of the time on business trips, Aaron didn't know whether or not Isaac was aware of Uncle Jacob's wishes for these properties. He did know that Isaac wanted both properties, most especially the island.

That evening Aaron planned to give Isaac a book he thought would be of interest. He also thought Isaac should see the letter, so he put it in an envelope in the book. He caught up to him at the club just as Isaac was getting out of his car. "Isaac, here's a book, also something for you to read later." It was getting late for their cocktail and dinner time. Since they had planned to meet their wives there, he felt they should move along.

Instead of tossing the book and envelope into his car, Isaac opened the envelope. "What's this?" Aaron turned and quickly responded. "This is a letter we both received. We can discuss it later." Isaac looked at the contents and stared at Aaron. "You believe someone from the trust company should be with us to sort this out. That's what you want!" Aaron was astounded. "Isaac, those are not my thoughts. I have only given you something to read which we can discuss later." "No," accused Isaac, "you want someone from the trust involved because you don't believe we can sort out the island and shore property the fishermen use! You don't believe we can do this by ourselves!"

Aaron couldn't believe it. He really didn't care whether they did it by themselves or included someone from the trust company. Isaac kept loudly accusing him of thoughts he didn't have. Aaron was concerned others nearby could hear. "Not now. Later, Isaac. We can talk about this later. Let's just move on and see if our wives have arrived." Aaron sighed, then turned around and slowly headed toward the clubhouse.

* * *

In this situation you make a comment or ask a question. The other person insists, or may even accuse you, of thoughts you don't have. No matter how much you try to clarify, you are not heard. Despite your denial, the other person holds onto an incorrect tenacious assumption and dogged belief about what you think, and will not be persuaded otherwise.

* * *

Jake was well trained as a mental health clinician. He interned at the Yale Medical Center and had been a senior clinician and supervisor at a major mental health center in California. He was familiar with complex psychotherapeutic and emergency situations. A few months earlier he had accepted a clinical position at a rural mental health service in a small town in Montana where his grandfather was a beloved country doctor. He adored his grandparents, had summered there for many years, and it had been his goal to return there permanently.

He worked hard those first few months. This morning he had just returned to the service after a week off. He went to the kitchen, poured a cup of coffee and offered one to Zeke, the administrator, the only other person in the room. Zeke shook his head to the coffee and asked Jake if he'd had a good vacation. "Yes, granddad and I got to see a rodeo." He began to continue but Zeke interrupted. "Jake, you're being sued. I was at the Board of Directors last night and told them our Yalie is being sued." Jake's mind started racing. Zeke continued. He named a local man who had telephoned him. "Harry said he was going to sue you and the clinic because you said he was paranoid." Jake knew who Harry was, but Harry was not his patient. Zeke went on. "Ada told Harry you said he was paranoid. So now he's going to sue us." Ada was his patient. Jake remembered that she had been upset that Harry had been making unseemly remarks about her when he saw her in town. She tried to avoid him, but found that impossible in this small town.

"Zeke, since I was on vacation did you pull the chart and read it?" Zeke hesitated then slowly shook his head. "I'll get it for you." Jake quickly returned with the chart and opened it to the notes. Jake pointed to the following written note. "Patient is angry at a man in town whom she feels makes unseemly remarks about her. She kept referring to him as paranoid. She said she can't seem to avoid him because the town is so small. She was not concerned that he would harm her, only that she felt he was a nuisance." Zeke looked at Jake. "Well, since Harry told us he will sue us, I told the Board."

Now Jake was furious. He knew he wouldn't call anyone by any such names. He certainly wouldn't diagnose anyone without seeing that person professionally. His administrator had not read the chart, had not waited to ask him about it, but had believed Harry and taken that belief to the Board as if it were true.

"Zeke, I know someone on the Board. If you don't clarify this with the Board, I'll go to the next meeting and talk with them myself. You call the chairperson and tell the facts. I'll talk with the Board member I know, and if you don't have this straightened out by the next meeting you can be sure I'll be there. Can't you see? Ada took her word, paranoid, attributed it to me, her therapist, to give it more credibility than if she had said it herself. Patients are known to do this."

A day later, George, a lawyer who occasionally offered legal advice to the mental health service, told Zeke that Harry had come into his office to have him sue Jake and the clinic. George already knew about this story which he had heard from Zeke. George listened to Harry then told him he doubted any psychotherapist would do what Ada had said, it would be very expensive to pursue, and it wasn't worth it because it was too soft a case. He told Harry he could consult another lawyer, but he didn't believe any lawyer would take it. Harry considered what George said and decided not to sue.

Two days later Jake talked with the Board member he knew who told him that the chairperson had heard from Zeke who clarified the situation including the fact that Harry had dropped the idea of a suit. Zeke never mentioned the situation again, nor did he apologize.

* * *

He said-she said situations are one of the most common types of assumption situations. Zeke listens to Harry who says thus and so, and Zeke believes him. Later he is surprised to hear an entirely different version from Jake. These situations are prevalent whether in health care or elsewhere. They can range from minor misunderstandings that need correction to major factual errors that can result in adverse actions that affect people's lives, such as in health care, but also elsewhere.

* * *

Kelsey walked into a telecommunication office in upstate New York. Standing in front of her were two people at the counter. The elderly man on the left was looking at Gerry, a clerk, who was in the back of the room focusing on some papers. The woman on the right was watching Rae who was taking a piece of paper that was coming out of the computer printer. Rae turned, looked at Kelsey and asked why she was there. "To discuss a bill." Gerry looked up from the back of the room and shouted at Kelsey. "You have to wait your turn," then refocused on her papers.

Kelsey was startled, then angry. Since Gerry and Kelsey had known each other for years, Kelsey couldn't believe Gerry would accuse her of not taking her turn. Rae glanced over at Gerry when Gerry shouted, then looked at Kelsey who responded as soon as the woman in front of her had taken the paper from Rae and left. "I was only answering your question. I don't jump lines!" Rae nodded and tried to calm Kelsey. "I know you wouldn't do that. Obviously Gerry misunderstood." "But I don't know how she could ever believe that of me," pleaded Kelsey. "I don't want a reputation that is not me. Will you please clarify this with Gerry when you get a chance?" Rae nodded. "Sure. Let's discuss your bill. I'll talk with her later."

* * *

In this type of situation you are there and completely ignored after an incorrect assumption is made and believed about something you said or did. You are not given an opportunity to respond. You may or may not be fortunate enough to have someone there whom you hope will later clarify the facts. Assumptions can be made very quickly. They can be automatic as if without conscious thought. If not verified they can also be incorrect, which may result in false beliefs and heightened emotions.

* * *

There were movie theaters in many small towns before television was available. These theaters showed newsreels before showing their movies, both of which were repeated for a few days. John told his mother, Alma, that he had seen his sister in one of these newsreels. Margie was a medical intern on ambulance duty in Toronto, Canada. "You should go see her," he said. "Dad would be pleased to know about this. You could tell him." His Dad was very ill in the hospital and his mother had been spending many hours by his bedside. John continued. "Some man was working on a very high chimney at the top of a tall factory building. The line that was holding him failed to hold him in place. He was trapped and couldn't go up or down. A rescue crew was trying to get him down. Margie was walking beside the ambulance at the foot of the building looking up at what was going on. She's in the film a few minutes. You can't miss her. She looks great. Go see it and tell Dad. He'd love it."

Alma was eager to see the newsreel. The next day she went to the theater, happened to see the owner, whom she knew well, so she told him she came to see the newsreel because John had told her Margie was in it. She did not plan to stay for the movie. "Come on in. I'm not going to charge you for just seeing the newsreel." This was an afternoon showing which gave her time to get to the hospital for a visit before her husband's supper. Indeed he perked up when she told him about the newsreel and how well Margie looked.

The next day Helen, a close friend, dropped by the house to get the latest news. She proceeded to tell Alma that a woman from the next town was criticizing her. This woman had seen her go into the theater and told Helen she couldn't understand why Alma would go to a movie when her husband was so ill in the hospital. "How could she?" grumbled this woman who had moved off while shaking her head. Helen had no answer because she didn't know the situation which was only clarified when she visited Alma the next day.

* * *

In this type of situation the meaning of your behavior is misinterpreted and may even be criticized. An incorrect assumption is made and told to others as if it were true. Because you are not there, you have no way of correcting it. The incorrect assumption which has become a dogged belief may be passed on to others. They may or may not accept what they hear. Unless someone tells you, you have no idea that this is going on. If never corrected, this incorrect belief about your behavior may be carried on for years.

* * *

Caleb was a spry ninety-year-old man who played golf three times a week with his golf buddies. His golf cart had a red flag on it which meant he could drive it on the golf course when others were required to use the cart paths. He said he needed the red flag because his knees sometimes bothered him, but denied that his arthritis had affected his golf game. He walked slowly, but his balance was good, and he could usually score close to his age of ninety, a good score for any amateur golfer.

He was furious at his seventy-five-year-old friend, Levi, who last winter had insisted on walking arm in arm with him over Levi's icy driveway to Caleb's car when Caleb visited. He kept complaining about this to his wife. "Levi treats me as if I'm an old man. I'm not an old man. I don't need anyone walking with me as if I'm an old man." "So why don't you tell him?" asked his wife. "No, I'll just hurt his feelings, maybe make him mad if I criticize him. You know Levi."

After hearing this more than she wanted, she finally remembered that a young friend of Levi's had slipped and fallen on ice, became unconscious for a few hours and had not realized it until he awoke in the hospital. The fall had resulted in a concussion and continuing memory problems. She reminded Caleb of this. "Maybe Levi is afraid this will happen to you. You know how much he cares about you. Maybe he's just remembering that accident which had nothing to do with age. Anyone can slip on ice." Caleb admitted he had forgotten this. He said that thought had never occurred to him.

Finally he asked Levi if he accompanied him to his car in the winter because he was afraid that what had happened to his friend who slipped on ice would happen to him. "Yes, Caleb, you know how close we've always been. I don't want anything to happen to you. That's the only reason I do it." Caleb melted. It surprised him how long he had carried these angry feelings about Levi's behavior, and that he had felt Levi would get angry if he tried to discuss it with him. Two incorrect assumptions had led to two dogged beliefs which were only corrected after some time had passed, and only after someone else offered other thoughts to consider.

* * *

In this situation you are the one making the incorrect assumptions. Your dogged beliefs that your assumptions are true prevent you from checking on their validity. They may even prevent you from entertaining other possible interpretations that might encourage you to verify whether or not your assumptions and beliefs are true.

ASSUMPTIONS CAN MISLEAD

These five stories include some of the most common types of situations with incorrect assumptions that can also be dogged beliefs. In the inheritance story you are there. Someone insists you have thoughts you don't have, and your attempt to clarify is ignored. The story where Zeke tells Jake he is being sued is a typical he said-she said situation. In some inaccurate he said-she said situations, the other person may never have an opportunity to state what is true. The story in the telecommunication office where an assumption is quickly made and you are not offered an opportunity to respond, is also fairly common. Incorrect assumptions can also be made about your behavior from someone who only observes you, such as in the story where Alma goes to see the newsreel that shows her daughter. You may never know about these assumptions unless someone tells you. In the final story about the elderly friends, Caleb and Levi, you make incorrect assumptions about someone else's thinking or behavior that you believe relates to you. If you don't realize it makes sense to talk with that person to verify whether or not your thinking is accurate, or obtain clarification by some other means, you may never know if your assumptions are correct. Whether problematic or not, firmly held incorrect assumptions can be dogged beliefs.

6. Automatic Assumptions Can Mislead

When we make an assumption we take something for granted. We accept it as fact. Many assumptions are automatic. We may not realize or even consider that our thoughts, feelings, or actions have come from assumptions that need verification.

* * *

Because of a meeting that morning, Andrea, the nursing supervisor, arrived late to the psychiatric unit. From conversations with Rhonda, the nurse in the medication room, she realized that none of the nursing staff had spent time with a new patient who had arrived at least an hour ago. This was surprising because it was expected that a staff member would talk with any new patients to orient them to the unit and begin to get to know them. Rhonda admitted she was afraid of this new admission, a tall, overweight man in rumpled clothes, who seemed to be in constant motion. She thought other staff members were also afraid of him even though they had no information to indicate that he would be a threat to anyone.

Andrea learned that his name was Walter. She recognized him as the tall patient with the black leather jacket and brown slacks, the only patient she didn't know. He was not actually pacing, but he was walking around with a serious expression and an unsteady gait. Though rumpled, his clothes looked clean. His red hair was neatly combed. He kept turning his head around as his eyes darted in different directions. His arms kept moving about. Should she feel afraid of him? She felt a little uneasy.

She went over to him. "Good morning, Walter. My name is Andrea. I'm the nursing supervisor." He quickly looked at her, then looked toward the door. He slowed down a little, but kept walking. He lifted one hand, then pushed back his hair. "Should I be afraid you'll hit me?" Walter slowed down some more, looked at her again, then shook his head. "No. I keep moving around like this because it's hard to stop. You see, I have a medical problem." He continued walking, but slowed down even more.

As they walked together he began to talk about his medical problem and his concern about having been admitted to the hospital. Andrea listened, then suggested they sit down over in the corner where it was quiet. "Are you able to do that? I'd like to get to know you and talk with you about what we might be able to do for you." "Yes," he said, "I can sit down, but I may not be able to stop moving about."

* * *

It's not unusual for any of us to make an automatic assumption that we are in danger when we feel unsafe. However, this is a psychiatric unit with staff who know the Orlando Model and are familiar with the behavior of psychiatric patients who need hospitalization. Walter had not done anything to indicate he would be aggressive and harmful. Even so, and even with their training in recognizing and verifying their assumptions, only the nursing supervisor was able to share her feelings with Walter as a way to begin a conversation and have him explain the meaning of his behavior. It is not always easy to recognize and clarify assumptions when they involve intense emotions, especially when we feel afraid for our safety. We accept such feelings as reasonable and may not realize they arise from automatic assumptions based on misinterpretations, in this situation of what was seen.

* * *

On October 12 and 13, 2009, television news headlined the following. A man was awakened at night by a noise in his bedroom. It was dark. He saw an outline of a person, grabbed his gun and fired. Unbeknownst to him, his fiancée had gotten up to go to the bathroom and was returning to bed. They were planning to marry the next day. His shot hit her in the chest and killed her.[1]

* * *

It is unclear whether or not they had discussed the fact that there had recently been burglars in the neighborhood, and that he planned to have his gun next to the bed. There was apparently no thought of checking to see if she were the person he saw. His reaction was based on a quick automatic assumption that his life was in danger, a misinterpretation of what he heard and what he saw.

* * *

Deer hunting in the fall is a passion for some in northern New England where I live. Because my Dad was a doctor, and he sometimes received venison as payment for services, I have been aware of this passion ever since I can remember. But tragedies are too often linked to this passion. A white flash or a movement in the bushes or woods can lead to a quick shot. Identification is not clear until after the gun is fired. Instead of a deer, a hunting partner or someone else has been wounded or killed. Once the white flash was a sheet on a clothesline in someone's yard. A woman was hanging out her laundry. She was killed outright. The automatic assumption here is based on expectation, it must be a deer, and wish, I want to be sure to get a deer this season. Yet again there is intense emotion with adrenalin flowing freely, this time emotion fueled by an expectation and a wish.

* * *

Susan Boyle, an amateur singer from Scotland, was an overnight sensation when she sang "I Dreamed a Dream" from *Les Miserables* on "Britain's Got Talent."[2] The initial belief was that she probably should not have been there. The audience laughed when Susan came on stage. She was a short, overweight, frizzy haired forty-seven-year-old woman dressed in plain clothes. Her movements were awkward. The audience chatted and were noisy with their restlessness. But when she began to sing they gasped, then became silent. Tears flowed. Her full, rich, sonorous voice rang throughout the hall. The judges sat spellbound. Listeners were speechless. Many felt her voice was as eloquent as any of the professionals who had sung that song in the show. When she finished, she received a standing ovation. A replay of some of her performance and her story remained in the media for days.

* * *

Until Susan sang many viewed her through the lens of a stereotype. Look at her. What's she doing here. Surely she can't sing well enough to be here. Stereotypical thinking is based on automatic assumptions that can lead us astray. Incorrect beliefs may not be changed unless we receive different information from what we have automatically expected. With her singing Susan offered new information to change any automatic incorrect belief and expectation about her.

* * *

Herman and Hannah live on fourteen acres of woods in northern New Hampshire amongst gorgeous beech, birch, and maple trees. Every few years they hire a tree service to cut limbs, or fell trees that might otherwise fall on their buildings or power lines. Craig comes, they all agree to the work, then Craig writes the work order and passes it on to the men who do the cutting.

Hannah was home the morning Brett and Jason arrived to do the work. An hour later the sound of their chain saws stopped. From the window Hannah noticed that the beech tree next to the barn had not been felled. She went outside.

She stopped beside Brett who was looking at the work order. "You probably know that the large beech tree beside the barn has to go." He didn't acknowledge her remark, so she suggested they walk over to the barn to look at the tree. He hesitated, then nodded, and followed her. She pointed out the dead limbs on the massive, still beautiful tree. "See," she said, "it has tape on the trunk. It needs to come down."

"It's not a designated tree." Brett briefly looked at Hannah, then turned, shook his head, and started walking back toward the truck. Hannah stayed right with him. "You saw the red tape on it. The tape is on it because it needs to come down. It is a designated tree." "Who put the tape on it?" He seemed annoyed. "I did," emphasized Hannah, "after my husband and I agreed that it needed to come down." "Well, we can't take it down."

Now Hannah was annoyed. They were headed into winter and the tree was not only dying, it was leaning toward the barn. She didn't want them to leave until they cut it down. They were almost at the truck. "Listen, why don't you come in and telephone Craig who agreed that this tree needed to come down when he was here discussing with us what needed to be cut." Brett suddenly stopped, turned and faced her. "Craig agreed to that tree?" "Yes. Craig agreed to it. If you don't cut it down now you'll just have to come back later and cut it down."

"Well, it's dead and unsafe for us to climb. We don't have the right equipment with us. We've done all we can do today." Brett spoke gruffly. Jason was already in the truck. Brett climbed in, started the engine, backed the truck around, and headed down the long driveway. Because Brett was curt, unusual for anyone from the tree service, and because it was important to have this tree felled before winter, Hannah went into the house and immediately telephoned Craig. What had happened became clear after Craig talked with Hannah and later with Brett.

Herman and Hannah had marked trees with red tapes. Craig accepted those tapes. To other trees he added yellow tapes with the printed name of the tree service in black. However, after Craig confirmed this work with Herman and Hannah, and before Brett and Jason arrived, the tree service learned that a woman for whom they recently did work had added her own tapes to trees after Craig left. The men who cut her trees didn't realize that Craig had not agreed to cutting all those limbs and trees the woman's tapes had indicated. She was billed for what she and Craig had discussed, not for all the work that was done. They realized the discrepancy when they talked amongst themselves after the work was done.

Even though the men doing the cutting are supposed to adhere to the work order, Craig's work orders don't always indicate specific trees. They may only refer to trees on a certain side of the property. Therefore sometimes the men in the past have asked Hannah or Herman what was to be cut. Not so on this day.

On this day the work order didn't match all the tree tapes. Brett knew about the situation with the woman, so he decided not to cut taped trees that weren't clearly noted in the work order. For Brett, designated trees were only those mentioned in the work order. For Hannah, designated trees were those marked with any tape, theirs or ones from the service.

In the work order Craig had not specifically mentioned the beech tree by the barn. So he told Brett he understood why he had not considered that tree as being included in the work. Craig also told him that all the tapes were legitimate. He explained that it is usual for Herman and Hannah to have different tapes than those of the service, because they use their own tapes to mark trees they're concerned about before he arrives. If needed, he adds tapes from the service. He also acknowledged to Brett that his work orders need to be more clear.

About a week later, two other men from the service came with the bucket truck and cut down the beautiful beech tree which really had to go. Now when Craig comes to mark their trees for cutting, Hannah insists he use the tree service tapes. And she reads his work order to see if it matches what the tapes indicate. She wants to prevent any similar misunderstandings.

* * *

This scenario is fairly common. The same word, in this case "designated," meant something quite different to the people who were using it. It never occurred to them that they were using the word differently. This situation might have been more difficult to resolve if no one had been home and if Hannah hadn't gone outside to inquire why the beech tree hadn't been cut down. Even then the situation wasn't clarified until Hannah telephoned Craig who followed up with Brett.

Sometimes people never realize they are not talking about the same thing. They may or may not become frustrated with each other. Their assumption that the other person understands them is not verified for accuracy because they may not even realize they are making an automatic assumption, let alone one that is incorrect.

* * *

These stories show how easy it is to automatically assume and act on such an assumption. The Susan Boyle story shows how seamlessly we can sometimes flow from our perceptions, in this case what was seen, to stereotypical thinking. Misunderstandings about what others mean by how they use words can sometimes mislead us, as noted in the tree service story. Actions from some quick, incorrect automatic assumptions, especially when one feels afraid, unsafe, and/or the adrenalin is flowing from an expectation or wish, can lead to misunderstandings or even deaths. In all these situations, usually we have not realized or considered that our thoughts or feelings have come from assumptions that needed verification.

7. Betrayed

It was September. Katie was a bright, eager, five-and-a-half-year-old first grade student who knew her letters, could do simple math, and loved to walk through the tall grass on her way to and from school. She lived in a small, rural, agricultural town. Everyone knew each other. There was no concern about letting even small kids walk to school if it were near. They had time to meet and greet each other and talk about whatever little kids share with each other. Many of them walk with older siblings.

This day she was not as cheerful as usual. She was walking home from school with her big brother whom she adored, and to whom she felt she could share most secrets. John looked down at his little sister. "How was school today?" Usually Katie would spill forth the day's events with obvious excitement. Not so today. Her head was down. She looked very sad. She didn't answer. She just shook her head. He was concerned. "What happened?" Her eyes began to fill with tears and she swallowed hard. "Please, tell me what happened." She began to tell her story as they neared and entered the tall grass.

"Miss Bristle gave us a test today. Just as I finished I heard her footsteps coming down the aisle. She leaned over and grabbed my paper. She put a red X on all my answers. I couldn't believe it. I thought I had all the answers right. She was furious. She told me I hadn't paid attention. Then she put a big F at the top. She said I should have known better. I tried to explain my answers, but she wouldn't listen. She kept yelling. She said I was flip. I kept trying to explain. She yelled louder and told me I should not interrupt. She slammed her ruler down on my desk and said she did not want to hear another word. She pushed my paper back at me, then headed for her desk." Katie was pouring out her story now. "I think all the kids were staring at me. I don't understand what I did wrong."

John was puzzled. He knew Katie was bright and a good student. "Tell me about the test. Tell me what you understood you were supposed to do."

Katie looked up at John, then down again. They were coming out of the tall grass now and headed toward the field. She hoped she'd finish before they reached their yard. "Well, there were ten questions on the test. Each question had a bunch of words on the left side. You were supposed to circle one word from the bunch of words that came closest to one word that was by itself on the right." She looked at him. He nodded. "So I did. I thought it was easy. I whipped through it. I picked the word closest to the one on the right. But she said all my answers were wrong!"

John encouraged her to go on. "Take one of the questions and explain how you answered and what she said about it."

"Okay. If it said red on the right, I picked out bed, the closest word. None of the other words had only one letter different. So I picked out the word that had only one letter different. But Miss Bristle said I should have picked out the same word. In the bunch of words was the same word. I hadn't noticed that because I wasn't looking for the same word. I was looking for the closest word. She pointed out red in the bunch and red on the right. I tried to tell her that wasn't the closest word, it was the same word. The directions didn't ask for the same word. The directions asked for the closest word. The closest is almost the same, but it is not the same. That's when she told me not to interrupt, that I was being flip. John, the same is the same. It is not the closest. You can be closest to something and not be the same." They were almost across the field. Her eyes began to fill with tears again. "I still don't understand why I was wrong." She hesitated. "John, what if I flunk first grade?"

"You won't flunk first grade. It was only one test. Your way of answering makes sense. It wasn't reasonable to ask for the closest then put in that bunch the same word. You have a good point. She just didn't want to hear it."

"Oh John, how am I going to get through first grade?" "You will, you will," he said as he reached down and took her hand as they crossed under the apple trees into their yard.

* * *

It was cold, this last week of August. Danny pulled her heavy warm sweater more tightly around her. She was nestled in the back seat of the car next to Max, her Golden Retriever. Her mother was driving her home after her two months at Camp Kenaki. She had just turned ten. She had been to this girls' camp for three years, and had made some very close friends. She would miss them but they'd stay in touch. They promised to write and meet at the winter reunion in Boston.

Danny and her family lived in Maine. These late summer days were often cold. She leaned closer to Max for his warmth. She was glad her mother had brought him. She had missed him. It was obvious he had missed her by his excitement when he saw her. She wanted to play and hike with him as much as possible before school started in a couple of weeks.

Now they were passing by the woods on the outskirts of town. They should be home in about an hour. She hoped Mark was around. He lived only a few houses away. They had always played together as kids. Their parents knew each other, and it was okay for them to come and go and play at either house.

She smiled as she thought about Mark, George, and Al. In winter she was goalie for them and the others that came over for hockey games on the lake. They also included her in their backyard football and baseball games. None of them went to summer camp. Even though they were a little older, they often asked her to join them. She never went by Danielle, her birth name. She insisted on being called Danny. She was one of the guys, and they accepted her.

She couldn't wait to get home. She looked up as they were turning onto Main Street. The street was quiet as they passed Bert's General Store. She'd have to get down there. He had a huge section of comic books. She didn't have much money. She'd blown it at the camp store. She couldn't buy any comic books now, but she had boxes of them at home.

She and the guys had been trading comics since they were much younger. All of them had good collections. They were somewhat competitive in their trading. It had become such a neighborhood activity that Lou, Al's older brother, had renovated an unused tool shed into a comic book business just down the road. Lou sold and traded comics with anyone who was interested. Mostly his customers were those in the neighborhood. But word had gotten around that Lou had collected a wide variety of comics in mint condition. He was fair. You could dicker with him such as six of your poorer copies for maybe four in mint condition. Superman and Batman were the rage. Outer space comics were becoming popular.

They turned into the driveway. As soon as she opened the door, Max bounded out of the car. Danny didn't see anyone outdoors.

It was time for lunch. So, after getting in the luggage, she had a sandwich and went to look for Mark. Max followed her.

Mark was in his yard stacking wood for the winter. He looked up with a big smile. "Welcome home. It's good to have you back. After I stack wood and get some lunch, how about taking some comics to Lou's and see what we can trade. It's supposed to rain tomorrow, so we might as well see what he's got to offer. We can sort out our collections when it rains and see if we want to trade any of ours with each other."

Danny was thrilled. She had hoped they would be doing something together this afternoon. "Great. I'll go see what I want to take to Lou's. Come on over after lunch." Mark nodded and waved as Danny turned and headed to her house with Max.

At the bottom of the stairs to the second floor she told Max to wait. He sat down and watched her run up the stairs. She skidded into her bedroom. Because her bed was high with a skirt around it, she had stored most of her comics in boxes under the bed. Those comics in mint condition she had stored in other boxes in her closet. She went down onto her knees and lifted up the skirt of her bed. Nothing there. This can't be, she thought. I know I stored most of them here. She got up and went over to her closet. She opened the door and looked under the clothes. No boxes there. She got a small ladder and climbed it to see what was on the shelf above the clothes rack. No comics there. What could have happened.

She ran out of the room, down the stairs, sailed by Max, and tore into the kitchen where her mother was baking cookies. "Mom, I can't find my comics. Do you know what happened to them?" Her mother hesitated, turned around and looked at her. "I gave them to the fair." Danny's heart skipped a beat. "What fair?" Her mother glanced at the oven then turned back and looked at her. "I gave them to the fair supporting the new wing at Oak Ridge Medical Center. You know they have a summer fair every year for the Medical Center."

Danny was dumbfounded. She couldn't believe it. She stared at her mother. She raised her voice. "Those were mine. I bought them or got them as a trade. They weren't yours. They didn't belong to you. I know you don't like things lying around, so I've always kept them under my bed and in my closet out of sight. Before I left I cleaned my room, including under the bed and the closet. There was no reason for you to go into my room." "Don't talk to me like that, Danielle." Her mother spoke sternly. They both stared at each other. Her mother turned and opened the oven door to check on the cookies.

Danny didn't want her mother to see the tears forming in her eyes. She turned and slowly walked out of the kitchen, then out of the house. Max followed her outdoors to their favorite stand of pine trees where they could see the ocean in the distance. She leaned against her favorite tree, then slowly slid to the ground. Max climbed into her lap. She hugged him as her tears fell silently onto her sweater. "How could she, Max, how could she."

* * *

Joan, a nursing manager, was on call that Sunday morning. She was paged to go to the hospital cafeteria. A little girl was sitting quietly at a table all by herself. A pink barrette held her brown hair back from her little round face. Soft curls fell just below her ears. It surprised Joan that the table was bare. There were no toys or food on the table in front of this tiny little girl. No one knew anything about her. The staff had thought her mother was in line getting breakfast, but there was no longer a line, and still there was no one with her.

Joan walked slowly over, made eye contact, and smiled. The little girl smiled shyly in return. "Hi, sweetie. What's your name?" A tiny voice responded. "Gina." "Where's your mommy?" There was no response. "How old are you?" She held up two little fingers. Joan noticed a small suitcase under the table by her feet. She pointed to it. "Is this yours?" Gina didn't respond.

Joan opened the suitcase and found a child's clean, neatly folded clothes. There were no toys, no books, and nothing that would identify her. "Are you hungry?" was answered by a small nod. Joan held out her arms. Gina eagerly reached out, then put her little arms tightly around Joan's neck and clasped Joan's waist with her little legs. Gina selected a carton of milk. She declined anything else. She seemed well nourished and healthy. But who could have left her this way without a trace.

Joan called the hospital social services. They contacted the hospital administrator on call, the police department, and the city social services. While Joan was involved with calls on her behalf, Gina paid attention with her big brown eyes, and answered questions with a nod or shake of her head. She made no other motions, no sounds. She continued to hold onto Joan with her tight grip. Eventually Joan was told to turn Gina over to a police officer who would take her to a case worker. The case worker was to take her to a foster home.

Joan described strapping Gina into the back seat of a police car as one of the most painful moments of her life. Gina had barely been out of her arms since she first saw her so alone in the cafeteria. She had been stoic and quiet during all this time. As soon as Joan put her in the police car with her little suitcase, Gina began to cry hysterically. Joan tried to talk to her soothingly and reassure her that everything would be all right. Gina would have none of it. She just looked at Joan with tear filled eyes, sobbing and reaching out to be picked up again. Joan finished fastening her in, gave her a final hug and kiss, shut the door, then turned around with tears now streaming down her face. It was the last time Joan ever saw her.[1]

* * *

Responding reasonably to someone includes knowing what that person thinks and feels about a situation when that information can be obtained. It may mean making an effort to encourage that person to share any opinions. Children are more vulnerable than adults who have had life experiences and challenges they have learned to meet. All children who are capable of stating their thoughts and feelings about situations deserve to be heard. Sometimes very ill people or little children may not be capable of offering information about situations that involve them. However, even then one should not make assumptions without careful thought about the effects of considered actions and possible solutions.

What solution would be best for that person? What solution would result in the least harm? What is the best way, the least harmful way, to reach that solution? Children and adults who are capable of stating their thoughts and feelings about situations that involve them may offer information or ideas that would not otherwise have been considered. It may feel like a betrayal when adults act contrary to their best interests and don't even consider their thoughts and feelings before the actions are taken.

Miss Bristle, Katie's first grade teacher, could not entertain the possibility that Katie might have a reasonable point to make. All Miss Bristle could see were incorrect answers according to the test requirements. Miss Bristle was thinking within the box, thinking automatically. The test required that the same word, viewed as the closest word, be taken from the bunch of words to match the word on the right. To Miss Bristle the same word was the closest word. To Katie closest was not the same, it was only almost the same. Instead of listening to what Katie was trying to say, Miss Bristle reprimanded her. Miss Bristle's lack of understanding and strident way of behaving were very painful to this little five-and-a-half-year-old. It was fortunate that John, her older brother, was there to support her. Even so, it is not surprising that Katie struggled with her tears and feared flunking first grade.

When Danny's mother decided to clean out Danny's room and dispose of the comic book collection when Danny was at summer camp, it appears that she never considered what it would mean to Danny. Danny knew her mother didn't like things lying around, so she had kept the collection out of sight. Removing the collection and giving it to the fair was her mother's need, not Danny's. In disposing of this collection when Danny was away, Danny's mother not only deprived her daughter of a major activity she had shared with her friends, she showed that she didn't even believe that it was important to talk with her about what that activity meant to her. No wonder Danny felt betrayed, and, like Katie, struggled with her tears.

Throughout my psychotherapy career I have heard mothers tell me they are going home to clean out their children's rooms, discard, or give away what they think their children no longer need, or what they don't want their children to continue to have. Sometimes they have already done so. They do not even consider including their children in this endeavor. Don't children have rights? Just imagine what would ensue if the children did this with their mother's things.

Gina was abandoned by someone who had been her caretaker. We have no idea who that person was. We don't know why Gina didn't respond to the question "Where's your mommy?" Does she not know? Was she told not to say anything? We just don't know. She is only two years old. She is sitting all by herself as she was presumably told to do. What is striking about this story is that the assumption was made that leaving Gina by herself in a hospital cafeteria was the only way to get her to someone who would care for her. Since it appears that the caretaker felt unable to continue to take care of her, why was there not a more reasonable way to get her to some other care? If it were to be foster care, why was not foster care pursued, finalized, then Gina given time to get to know her new caretakers before the final placement? One can go to social services and discuss such situations. This situation to this little girl was a supreme abandonment.

It appears that these adults didn't realize they were acting on automatic assumptions that left out children whose feelings and thoughts deserved to be considered. It is especially poignant when children are betrayed by adults whose actions result in such heartache.

8. Now Will You Listen

I was on call for the mental health service that hot summer night. It was still light outside, about 7:30 p.m. I picked up the phone after the first ring. The hospital emergency room nurse said a woman had just been brought in by the state police. Could I come and see her? I told her I'd be there in about fifteen minutes. My mind was busy as I drove to the hospital. I was puzzled that the state police had brought someone to the emergency room. Rarely are they involved with our local patients.

The staff looked up as the door swished behind me. A nurse who knew me came over and walked with me down the hall toward the room where they had put this woman. She told me they didn't know anything about her circumstances. She was twenty-three, her name was Louise, but she preferred to be called Lou. As required, a doctor had briefly evaluated her and had determined that she was essentially physically healthy. I recognized that the tall policeman standing near her room was state police by his uniform. It flashed through my mind that I was surprised he was here. I prefer to have patients tell their stories first, so I told him I was from the mental health service, would talk with her, and headed toward the room. He looked down at me, nodded, turned around, reached out and opened the door. I went in.

A thin woman in light tan wrinkled pants and a lightweight long sleeved partly opened blue shirt was sitting on the examining table. The sheet under her was wrinkled. Another sheet partly covered her lap. She looked disheveled. Her uncombed shoulder length brown hair covered some of her face. Her head was down. She looked up as I walked in. She had been crying and she was dabbing her eyes with some tissues. She shoved her hair away from her face. I told her who I was, and added that I was there to help her in any way I could. I said I knew her name was Louise, but I heard that she preferred Lou. She nodded as I pulled over a chair and sat down in front of her.

She was still looking at me, so I asked her what happened. She immediately responded. "My roommate and I argued." Still not knowing why the state police was involved, I encouraged her to go on. It seemed clear that she needed someone who would really listen, so I said little, other than asking questions to be sure I understood what she was saying. At first she talked haltingly. She kept looking carefully at me to be sure I was following her. When I glanced at the clock, she stopped talking. She seemed sensitive to any diversion. But she had stopped crying and was making consistent eye contact. I realized it was important for me to keep eye contact with her. As I focused on what she was saying, and indicated I understood how she felt, she continued with her story and offered more and more detail.

Lou and her roommate lived a couple towns away. They usually got along, but sometimes they argued. When that happened, Lou said she felt her roommate didn't care about her. She would accuse her roommate of not listening and not caring. Her roommate said that was not true. Not to agree about something didn't mean she wasn't listening or that she didn't care.

This led to our having a long conversation about how one can disagree but still care. Finally Lou got the point when she realized she sometimes feels that way. She said she always cares about her roommate even when she doesn't agree with her. She admitted she can easily become hurt and take things personally. She said she came from a chaotic childhood where she felt her parents didn't care. She was aware those feelings had followed her into other relationships.

In the course of our conversation she acknowledged she was one of our clinic patients. She liked her therapist who had helped her figure out some of what we were talking about. Her next appointment with her therapist was tomorrow morning, and she was looking forward to seeing her. She not only looked better, she acknowledged she was feeling better. She had no delusions or hallucinations. She was not on any medications and denied having any at home. She was coherent and knew the approximate time. She clearly knew where she was. She seemed comforted that people were concerned and taking care of her.

I still didn't know how the state policeman got involved. So I asked her what happened to result in his bringing her to the emergency room. She referred to a major highway in the next town, and said he had picked her up there. She had been wandering, not paying attention, and he stopped to talk with her because she was too far out in one of the lanes. She didn't tell him she was upset and had walked out on her roommate. "But I think he figured I was upset because I had trouble talking with him. I couldn't seem to answer his questions. I kept mixing up my words, or I just didn't say anything. He told me he wanted to bring me to the hospital because he didn't want to leave me there. He said he was worried about me, and wondered if I needed to be in a hospital." "To bring you here, was that okay with you?" I asked as I kept looking at her. "Oh yes. I've been here before. I've been to the hospital in Concord, too."

Further conversation revealed that she had recently been taken to the state psychiatric hospital because she had been suicidal. "Do you feel suicidal now?" "No," she said. "I'm not suicidal. I just felt abandoned and confused." She paused. "I just want to keep my appointment tomorrow morning with my therapist." She also wanted to return home. She felt she had misunderstood her roommate. She had walked out without telling her where she was going. She thought her roommate might be worried about her, because she'd been worried when she had walked out before.

I offered her the possibility of talking with her roommate by phone. She said no, she just wanted to return home. She again reassured me she wasn't suicidal, and she didn't need to be in any hospital. She just wanted to go home and see her therapist in the morning. She added that she felt our conversation had been helpful, that she had been able to rethink things. Clearly she looked better and sounded better. I told her I'd ask the state policeman if he'd drive her home. She agreed to the plan.

When I asked him if he'd drive her home, he shook his head in disbelief. "You're not going to commit her to the state hospital? We took her down there recently. Do you know that she was wandering in the highway and could have been hit? Do you know that she's been suicidal before?" He sounded annoyed.

I acknowledged that I knew the information he had just mentioned. I told him I realized she is very sensitive, but she and I had talked about what she was going through. I stated that she has a good relationship with her roommate, that she has an appointment with her therapist in the morning, and she wants to keep that appointment. I added that she is not suicidal now. He sighed and shook his head again. "Are you sure?" "Yes," I said with emphasis,

"I'm sure. Will you drive her home? She needs a ride home." He paused, looked away as if he were thinking, sighed, turned his head back in my direction, looked down at me, and paused again. "I'll take her home," he said with what sounded like resignation. "Thanks," I said, "she'll appreciate it. I will too." He nodded.

I gave a brief summary to the emergency room nurse and signed off. On my drive home I realized that the state policeman may have been expecting to drive her to the state psychiatric hospital in Concord that evening. As a state policeman he may have been on his way to Concord when he saw her. He had picked her up north of the hospital, and Concord is an hour south. Also, since he knew she was recently there because of suicidal thinking, he may have wondered if he, the local police, or sheriff's department might be called later if I were incorrect. Her wandering on the highway may have made him think she was seriously suicidal again. If he had thought he would be taking her to the hospital on a commitment, that would not have been surprising. If he had been on his way to Concord anyway, a trip with her would have spared the local police or sheriff's department from arranging transportation for her.

I heard no more from this situation that night. Lou kept her appointment at the mental health clinic the following morning. Her therapist acknowledged that Lou is sensitive to hurts and tends to feel people take her for granted. She was pleased that Lou had adequately sorted through her feelings so she did not have to return to the psychiatric hospital in Concord.

* * *

On November 28, 2007, about a month before the New Hampshire presidential primaries, Leeland Eisenberg, age forty-six, entered Hillary Clinton's Rochester, New Hampshire, campaign office about 1:00 p.m. and held five people hostage. Local and national news followed the events for some five hours until the situation was resolved. Nearby stores hastily closed, streets in the vicinity were blocked off, police covered the perimeter, people gathered as close as they were allowed, and a negotiator began to talk with Leeland by phone.

The week before, citing irreconcilable differences, Leeland's wife had filed for divorce. He had a history of alcohol and drug abuse, and she said she was a victim of his verbal abuse. Leeland was a troubled man with a painful background. In the early 1980s he was homeless. To psychologically deal with having a violent alcoholic father and the death of his mother, in 2002 he sought refuge at a Catholic parish. He was one of 541 victims of the clergy sexual abuse scandal who received payments in the 2003 settlement with the Roman Catholic Archdiocese of Boston. Because of his various struggles, he was known to police and mental health services.

That morning his stepson said Leeland asked him where he could buy road flares. He told his stepson to watch the news that day. That afternoon Leeland walked into the campaign headquarters. He was neatly dressed in gray slacks, a white dress shirt, and a red tie. He had bought the flares, duct taped them to himself, and had a mock detonator. With this contraption attached to his clothes, it appeared he had a bomb. He said he wanted to talk with Hillary Clinton because he wanted help and couldn't get anyone to help him. He talked about one of the Clinton campaign commercials. It featured a New Yorker telling how Clinton had helped his son get a bone marrow transplant that their insurance would not cover. Because of this ad, Leeland thought she could help him.

His stepson said Leeland had been turned away from some medical facilities. He knew Leeland had been refused some medication because he didn't have insurance. His family said he had been turned down for mental health treatment because of lack of insurance. When Leeland was in the campaign office he called one of the major television stations and said he wanted to talk with Clinton by phone about getting psychiatric care that he could not afford.

Throughout the ordeal Leeland told his hostages he was just sick and desperate. He told them that he was not going to hurt anyone. He just wanted help. He immediately let one woman with a baby leave the building. When he was on the phone with the negotiator, the negotiator indicated they wanted to help him. When he finally came out, they arrested him and learned that his bomb was a fake.

His stepson believed this was an act of desperation to get some help. The hostages said Leeland had told them that he didn't want to hurt anyone. Later Leeland said he expected to be shot when he came out the door. He reemphasized that he never had any intention of harming anyone. If he had been shot, he said he was willing to sacrifice himself to get out the message of how one can be turned away from services one needs. If necessary, he felt he was willing to sacrifice himself just to get out the message.[1]

* * *

I was on call for the mental health service and reading a book when the ringing phone startled me. I glanced up. It was winter, 9:38 p.m., and pitch black outside. I picked up the phone and answered with "Hello." A woman acknowledged me with "Hi" followed by my name. "This is Glenna at the hospital." I knew she was the evening switchboard operator. Those folks have our on call schedule.

"I have someone on the other line I'd like to switch over to you. She wants to talk with mental health on call." "Okay, thanks." I heard a click, then Glenna said, "Go ahead."

I identified myself by name adding that I was the mental health person on call. A woman's voice immediately responded. "I've taken all my pills." My heart skipped a beat.

"What were the pills?" She answered with barely a pause. "I don't know. They're for my depression." "How many do you think you took?" Again she didn't hesitate. "I don't know. The bottle was partly filled." I asked her name which she readily told me. I asked her where she was. "I don't know." So I followed it with "what phone are you using?" Again she immediately answered. "I'm at a pay phone." This was before cell phones. I grew up in this area and had been back here for a number of years. But I had no idea where the pay phones were. My priority was to get her to the emergency room. I urgently needed more information, so I continued with more questions.

I needed to know where she lived, and if there might be someone there who could help us. So I asked her what town she lived in, was she currently a patient at our clinic, and was there someone at her home who knew she had been coming to the clinic. She gave me the name of her town, acknowledged that she was one of our current patients, and said she lived with her parents who knew she had been seeing us. She gave me her home phone number as soon as I requested it. This information offered me some relief. She lived in a rural town where houses can be difficult to find at night. At least I could call and talk with her parents. I needed their help.

I was aware she had been alert enough to know she should call the hospital to get to mental health on call, rather than calling 911 should she need our emergency service outside clinic hours. I noted that she had not been slurring, had not hesitated about answering my questions, and she had remained coherent. Time was on our side. Even so, she had not been able to answer specific questions about the medication, so I still felt an urgency to get her to the emergency room.

"How close to home are you?" Her voice was still strong as she said, "About ten minutes." Since I had recognized the name of her home town, I knew she was probably close to an hour away from the hospital and our emergency vehicles. But I couldn't tell them where she was.

"How did you get to the pay phone?" Another quick answer, "My car." I asked if she thought her parents could drive her to the hospital emergency room. "My Dad can." Good. She was easily and readily responding to me and to a possible plan. She acknowledged that her car keys were in her pocket. I had her tell me she could feel them there.

"I'm going to call your Dad and tell him to drive you to the emergency room. I'll call the emergency room and tell them you're on your way. You need to get in your car right now and drive home. Can you do that?" She responded with a firm "Yes." "Good, we'll be out looking for you if you don't get right home. Now get in your car and drive home," I said as firmly as I could. "Okay," she said. I heard the phone click, then silence.

I called her Dad who was very concerned and willing to drive her to the hospital. He knew the emergency room entrance. He understood that he needed to be ready to take her there just as soon as she reached home. He said he'd look for her and they would go right in. He acknowledged that I would be calling the emergency room, and they would be waiting for her. I gave him my home phone and told him to call me if she wasn't home in about ten minutes. He said he would.

Then I called the emergency room with the relevant details. I talked with a nurse I knew well, and she acknowledged my information. She promised me she would telephone me if this patient and her Dad had not arrived within the hour. Though it wasn't necessary, someone in the emergency room called later and reassured me that she had arrived.

Early next morning I learned that her therapist had been told about the evening's events from a nurse who had called from the hospital. The patient had been admitted overnight. She was fine, but needed a follow-up this morning. Her therapist had already left to see her.

* * *

Lou, Leeland, and the woman who took all her pills were feeling various degrees of hopelessness. Though they came from different circumstances, they had reached almost the end of their coping abilities. They were desperate to be heard, to be helped, and to get the caring they needed. Lou aimlessly wandered about on a major highway, flirting with disaster. When people showed concern, caring, and listened to her she became able to sort through her immediate issues, and to feel better. Leeland made a desperate attempt to be heard, and to be helped. His help came only after the authorities took over. Unfortunately he did not receive the help he needed when he sought it earlier.

The woman who took all her pills feared losing her life. I don't know what prompted her to take the pills. But at least she was eager to undo what she had done. She willingly responded to help. I didn't know her parents, but her Dad seemed appropriately concerned and worried when I talked with him by phone.

We need to feel there is someone who will listen, someone who will care. But there are times when we may feel that no one cares. If these feelings lead to desperate actions such as those here, the message is clear: Now will you listen.

9. The Need to be Heard

I've heard or read different versions of this story, all of which claim to be true. This version stays with its major theme and may or may not be similar to other renditions. The story takes place in a large well known toy store.

* * *

It is the week before Christmas. Two little girls have been told by their mothers that they can each pick out their very own, very special doll as a Christmas present. The third floor of this toy store has many shelves with all kinds of dolls. The expensive dolls are on one side of the store. Those dolls are made with costly materials. Many offer anywhere from one to five functions. The highest priced have all five functions. For each of those dolls, once you find the right place to press or the correct string to pull, the doll will wet, cry, laugh, talk, or blink. There are lower priced dolls made with lower cost materials that have none of these functions. They are on the other side of the store.

The mothers with their daughters are taking the escalator to the third floor. Both mothers are familiar with the store. They know the layout of the doll floor.

Mrs. McMartin is dressed in a well tailored tan suede jacket, dark brown wool slacks, and matching winter boots. She is with Maria, her six-year-old daughter, who is dressed in a gray wool jacket, purple winter slacks, and gray boots. Maria is wide eyed as the escalator is nearing the third floor. She can't believe all the dolls she begins to see.

Mrs. Toby and Tammy, her six-year-old daughter, are not dressed in expensive clothes. Their clothes are clean, but obviously worn. Both are wearing faded navy corduroy slacks. Mrs. Toby's tan coat cuffs are frayed. Tammy's faded dark green jacket is missing a button. Her cuffs are torn, but held together by velcro. She and her mother have taken the escalator just behind Mrs. McMartin and Maria. Tammy's eyes open wide as she and her mother near the top of the escalator at the doll floor. She, too, is almost overwhelmed with all the beautiful dolls that slowly come into view. The dolls are standing in their opened boxes with tissue lightly around them.

Maria eagerly looks up at her mother. "Can I have a doll that wets, cries, and laughs?" Mrs. McMartin chuckles and looks down at her. "You can have a doll that does all those things and, if you wish, you can choose one that also talks and blinks. You can choose any doll you want." As they reach the third floor her mother takes her hand. They step off the escalator and turn left toward the expensive dolls.

Since Tammy and her mother are riding up the escalator just behind Mrs. McMartin and Maria, Tammy hears their conversation. She looks up at her mother and asks, "Can I have a doll that cries, laughs, and talks?" Her mother pauses and looks down at her. "You can get a better doll. You can have a doll that listens." She takes her hand as they reach the third floor. They step off the escalator and turn right toward the less expensive dolls.

Maria takes some time to decide on her doll. She finally decides on a girl doll with a blond ponytail, a shiny bright red skirt and green jacket with a matching shiny red and green headband. She takes the doll, sees the strings, and tries to figure out their functions. She's supposed to push on her somewhere to get her to wet, but can't figure that out. Her mother says the doll has to drink water before she can wet and tells her they can do that at home. Maria understands, stops pulling on the strings and puts the doll back into the box. Her mother takes the box, pulls the tissue over the doll, and they head toward a cashier.

Maria quietly follows her mother as her mother pays for her doll that has remained in the box. The cashier puts the box and receipt into a plastic bag, which she gives to Mrs. McMartin. Maria carries the bag by its handle as they head toward the escalator.

Tammy's eyes have not stopped moving as she walks around and looks over all the beautiful dolls. Their clothes are made of soft materials in more subdued colors than the higher priced dolls. She knows she wants a doll who will listen. Which one? She spies a girl doll with curly brown hair and bright blue eyes. The doll seems to be looking at her. The doll has on a light blue sweater, matching blue sweat pants, and little white sneakers. A red plaid blanket is partly around her. Tammy reaches out and takes the doll with her blanket out of the box. As she does this, she starts talking softly to her. The doll continues to look at her. Tammy carefully covers her with the blanket, then cradles her over her shoulder, still talking to her. Her mother takes the empty box, looks down at Tammy who is still busily talking to her doll, lightly taps her shoulder to get her attention and motions the way to another cashier.

Tammy is still earnestly talking to and cradling her doll as she and her mother go to their cashier with the empty box. The cashier smiles when she sees the little girl busily whispering to a doll carefully covered with a red plaid blanket. Mrs. Toby quietly pays. The cashier nods. Tammy barely notices them as she and her doll follow her mother through the cashier's aisle, and head back to the escalator. Mrs. Toby's plastic bag has the empty box and the receipt. Tammy tightly hugs her doll as she catches up to her.

* * *

Willie began talking nonstop when he was around three. Before that he didn't talk much. His parents weren't worried that he mostly nodded or shook his head to a question, rather than answering with words. He always seemed to be listening. He figured out things. If his little train got stuck behind the couch he'd back it up, squiggle it around, and move it different ways until it was free. He loved to look at his books with the pictures. He welcomed anyone reading to him, especially when they asked him to point out the man with the red hat or the lion or the big tree with the swing. Oh yes, maybe he didn't say many words then, but he was very active and certainly bright.

After he turned three he'd quickly put up three little fingers when asked his age. And my, oh my, how he would talk. He'd talk about anything and everything. He has very loving, caring, responsible parents and grandparents. They answer his questions, patiently listen to his monologues, and clarify if he misunderstands something. His grandmother, who has extraordinary patience, would sometimes feel flooded by his constant chatter if she were alone with him for a number of hours during these early talkative years.

During the week his mother spends much time alone with him. When he started talking so much, it didn't take long for her to sometimes feel overwhelmed too, especially if he kept asking many questions and expected answers. She learned that when she needed some space, whether or not she had other things to do, he'd accept her telling him she needed quiet time.

"Willie," she'd say, "I need some quiet time now. You can play with your toys by yourself." She'd go to the table, sit down, pick up the mail and read it. Or she'd go and do things in the kitchen, all the while keeping track of where he was and what he was doing. She found this worked well. He'd look up, notice where she was, and continue to play. And he would continue talking. When he was moving his train he'd talk about what it was doing and what he wanted it to do. When he was putting together puzzles with animal pieces he might say, "horse goes there," or "oops, not right." He'd usually laugh if his stack of wood blocks fell down. He also enjoyed knocking them down.

Out loud he talked about all sorts of things. She'd hear him mention a stream of thoughts that crossed his mind. When he was hungry he'd go to the cupboard, get out the box of crackers, and take a cracker, all the while telling her why he was there and what he was doing. Next thing, he'd be with his little cars. "Vroom, vroom," he'd say as he moved them around the furniture, around the blocks, around the train, around the room, "vroom, vroom." His mother realized he was taking in everything. His parents and grandparents were continually amazed at his ever growing vocabulary. Whether he was with other people or by himself, it seemed that his mind was very busy figuring things out, sorting things out, asking questions to check things out, and soaking in as much as possible of what was going on around him including activities that interested him.

* * *

Each August I join my family at our local hospital street fair as a volunteer at the booth that sells tickets for rides. Some rides are suitable for small children. My favorite shift is 10:00 a.m. to 1:00 p.m. because that's when the little children come with their parents. When it's not busy I talk with them. "How old are you?" I say to the younger of two girls. "I'm three," she says while intently looking at me with her chin resting on the edge of the ticket counter. The older girl just behind her stops and thinks, catches my eye, and states "I'm four-and-three-quarters." She wants to be sure she is included. "Wow," I say as I nod and look at each of them. Their mother smiles down at them, then pays for their tickets.

Others listen as their parents discuss the rides with me. The children want to know which of the rides they can take. The parents are good about explaining the rides and being sure their children get the rides they want. Sometimes the parents will give their children the money for the tickets and tell them to give it to me. The children are quiet and attentive as I carefully count the money out loud, then put the change and tickets into their little hands. They keep the tickets and pass the change back to their parents. Responding to my wave, they wave a quick good-bye. Their faces are intent as they scurry around the booth toward the rides.

I comment and ask about the words or pictures on their tee shirts. "You like the Red Sox?" I ask a little boy in dungarees who is wearing a Red Sox tee shirt. He gives me a big nod. "Do you play baseball?" He gives me another big nod. Then he lets loose. "You know what, I won a bear today." He is now leaning on one arm at the edge of the ticket counter. With his free hand he lifts up a tan bear from below the counter and shows it to me. "He's beautiful," I comment. "Where did you get him?" He points to another booth. "Throwing bean bags over there. I have another bear like him at home." His Dad, who has been standing behind him, reaches out to touch him to attract his attention. Because there is no line I wave his Dad away. "Let him finish," I tell his Dad who acknowledges my comment by putting his arm down, smiling, and rolling his eyes as if to say here we go again. I grin back at Dad and refocus on the little boy who has continued his story while still looking at me. When he finally stops I exclaim that I've enjoyed talking with him, hearing about his bears, and congratulate him on winning this beautiful bear. "Enjoy the rides," I say as he nods, grins, then turns and runs around the booth toward the rides.

* * *

As the clinical director of a mental health service I supervised staff on their clinical work. One day one of the senior clinicians grabbed my arm and started describing a situation as I was walking down the hall. I was already late on the way to my office to see a patient. I knew this clinician well. She was experienced and making sense, so I interrupted and said "You don't need to tell me this. I trust your judgment." Immediately she responded with intensity. "I need you to hear this. I want to know what you think."

That brought me up short. Her tone as well as what she said emphasized that she needed to tell me her thoughts and hear my response right then. I stayed, listened, and supported her thinking. I apologized to my patient for being ten minutes late. He agreed to stay an extra ten minutes to make up the time. He, too, deserved his time in which to be heard.

* * *

Carmella's first psychotherapy appointment was on a bitterly cold winter day. I met her in the waiting room and showed her the way to my office. She was wearing a heavy long tan winter coat, a navy wool hat pulled way down over her ears, matching navy wool mittens, and dark brown fleeced lined winter boots. As she came into the office I told her she could use the wooden hanger and hooks on the back of the door to hang her coat and hat. With a serious expression, she nodded. Very slowly she took off her mittens, folded them, and put them in one of her coat pockets. In a similar slow manner she removed her hat, folded it and put it in the other pocket. She took much time unbuttoning each of four coat buttons. Then, continuing as before, she took one arm out of her coat, then the other. She turned around, took the hanger, carefully put the coat on it, hung the hanger on the hook, and turned around again. I motioned to a chair. In the same prolonged manner she went to it and sat down. I felt I was watching a movie in slow motion. Removing these clothes had taken about five minutes.

Her face was pale from the cold, her cheeks slightly red. Her short, black, curly hair was rumpled from taking off her hat. Her navy wool slacks and purple sweater were neat and clean. She appeared to be of average height and weight. The paperwork she had filled out indicated no medical problems, no previous treatment for mental illness, and she was not taking any medications. She had written "depression" as a reason for coming.

I looked up from the paperwork. "What prompts your coming for an appointment?" She blinked, paused, then said, "My mother told me to come." "Do you feel you need to come here?" She hesitated then answered, "I don't know." Her words were spoken slowly and softly. It was hard to hear her.

"Your paper says depression." Carmella was looking toward the window. "Do you think you're depressed?" She turned and looked back toward me. "My mother thinks so." "And do you think so?" I said as she continued looking at me. There was a long pause. "That's what my mother said." Her expression had been serious ever since I saw her in the waiting room. It had not changed. When I asked if she agreed with her mother, she didn't answer. She seemed baffled that I asked her opinion when she had already told me what her mother thought, as if that were sufficient. She had continued to talk slowly and softly.

"How do you feel about being here?" Since she had offered no views of her own, I felt it was very important to see how she'd answer. "Okay," she responded. "Can you tell me more about yourself, such as what you do, what your days are like?" She did not respond to this question or to any other open ended questions. So I stayed with questions that asked for specific facts. She had completed high school. She used to work in a small general store, but lost her job when the business failed. She wanted to work in a library. She liked to read, mostly mystery or romance. She was twenty-eight, had no boyfriends, and couldn't think of anyone who was ever her boyfriend. She never had a close friend and couldn't name any friends now. She was an only child and had always lived with her parents. Her mother did not work. Her father owned a small service station where he worked many hours, including weekends. He sold gas, repaired vehicles, and was on call to assist people on the road with their vehicles, as needed. Sometimes she'd drive over and visit with him.

Occasionally Carmella and her mother went to the movies. I asked what they had seen and when. She mentioned a movie they had seen the previous week. "Did you like it?" She answered with ease, "My mother thought it was good." "And you?" I looked at her hoping for her opinion. Yet again, no answer about what she thought. No opinions of her own, only those of her mother. She had not offered any spontaneous thoughts during this visit. Her history indicated that she was reasonably bright and had been able to handle a job.

It was striking that whenever I asked for her thoughts she'd always refer to her mother, such as, "My mother thinks . . ." or, "My mother says . . . ." It appeared that she didn't realize she was constantly deferring to her mother's views. She responded to these questions as if her answers were reasonable. If I told her I was asking for her opinion she lowered her head and seemed distressed, as if I were criticizing her. She'd respond with silence or "I don't know" in a lowered voice.

I stopped pressing for her opinions. If this first visit made her too anxious, she might not return. She had answered many factual questions slowly, but with no apparent distress. She took her little dog for a walk, so she was getting outdoors and getting exercise. She was sleeping adequately, her diet was reasonable, and she denied any significant symptoms other than depression. She agreed to return the following week and easily accepted the appointment card with its relevant information.

Then as slowly as when she entered, Carmella got up, turned, and put the appointment card in one of her coat pockets. She took the coat off the hanger. With the same slow speed as before, she slowly put her left arm into her coat, then the right. She pulled the coat higher so it fit better on her shoulders. Then she slowly buttoned the four buttons. She took the hat from the pocket, unfolded it, and slowly put it on, covering her ears. She took the gloves from the other pocket and put them in her left hand. With her right hand she reached for the door and opened it. She turned around, looked at me, said "Bye" with a serious expression, then left. She had taken another five minutes putting her clothes back on. I was now late for my next appointment and realized I needed to allow more time for her to remove and put on her clothes. I had never seen anyone at an office visit take so long doing this.

Her psychotherapy visits continued weekly for a few months. She always came on time. For the first few visits she took about the same length of time to take off and put on her coat, hat, and mittens as she had at the first visit. We talked about her childhood, her life, and her interests. When she answered "My mother says . . ." to questions asking for her opinion, I now followed up with "Do you agree with your mother?" She'd pause and say "Yes." She'd deny having thoughts that were different. Her mood did not remarkably change. But after a couple weeks she said she felt she had more energy.

Since Carmella took her dog for walks I'd ask her to describe those walks. I'd ask her anything that might encourage her to offer thoughts of her own. She was able to talk more freely about her visits with her dad at the gas station than about her time with her mother. When I made sure to look at her and listen carefully, she would talk without a pause. Her sentences were short, without much description. When she thought I wasn't listening, she'd immediately slow down or stop until she felt sure that I was hearing her. It was also important to her that I agreed with her opinions when it was appropriate to do so. She desperately needed support for thoughts of her own. Her sentences became longer with more description as the weeks moved on. She was also using up less time with her coat, hat, and mittens.

As her therapy progressed she slowly began to admit that she was becoming aware of having various opinions that were different from those of her mother. She wouldn't tell her mother, but she'd expand on them with me. Then, cautiously and carefully, she began to tell her mother when and in what ways she thought differently. At first it was about movies or television they both saw. Then it was about what her mother felt she should do, such as trying to get a job in a grocery store when she wanted a library job. Next it was about going by herself to buy a couple sweaters she had seen advertised. She had her own money. She wanted to decide and to make the purchase on her own. Previously, her mother had always gone with her. Carmella said her mother at first seemed surprised when she openly disagreed. But Carmella was pleased that her mother did listen. They were even able to disagree and stay on friendly terms. She was especially pleased that her mother supported her going on her own to decide and to purchase the sweaters.

Her relationship with her father had seemed supportive. It appeared even more so as her therapy progressed. She spent more time visiting with him at his gas station. She sometimes stayed to handle the cash register. She spontaneously mentioned that he appreciated this help from her. If she could say he appreciated her help, maybe she was beginning to appreciate herself.

By her last appointment she no longer felt depressed. She was able to bring in her agenda without any prompting from me. Her mood was lighter. She seemed more engaged in what she chose to discuss. The time she now took taking off and putting on her winter clothes was not noticeable. Within less than a minute she'd come in, stuff her mittens and hat into her pockets and hang up her coat. She'd sit down and start talking as soon as I asked how she was. She was able to leave as easily and as swiftly. The difference coming and going was truly remarkable.

Carmella understood she could return for more appointments if she felt the need. She stated that she now felt a confidence she had never felt, she had more energy and interest in life, and she had come to value her own thoughts and enjoyed standing up for her own opinions. Since she enjoyed reading and hoped to get a library job, she was planning to join a reading group at the library where she hoped to make friends. She smiled and nodded as she left after her last appointment. I never heard from her again.

* * *

These stories highlight how essential to our lives is the need to be heard. As babies we need our caretakers to hear and adequately respond to however we express our physical and emotional needs, or we literally fail to thrive. As soon as we are able, we need to hear ourselves think to know more clearly what we think and feel and to sort it all out. Children with caring, responsible adults clearly show this. Without hesitation, Tammy is thrilled to get a doll who listens. Her nonstop chatter continues on through the cashier aisle. Once Willie finds words, he shows us this need and more. Out loud he sorts out what he is thinking, what he is doing, and how to do it. He also learns from his parents and grandparents who willingly answer his numerous questions and correct his misunderstandings. They listen to understand, and they respond appropriately. When his mother needs quiet time, he is able to continue his chatter by himself. As children grow older they sometimes have imaginary playmates with whom they carry on conversations. This also helps them sort out their numerous thoughts and feelings.

The staff member at the mental health service seeks further support and advice about a situation that concerns her. That, too, shows another way we need to be heard. Sometimes we need someone else to hear us sort through problematic situations. It can be helpful and appropriate to seek such support.

In order to develop a unique and stable identity, we need others to understand and appreciate what we uniquely think and feel. Willie and the children at the hospital street fair show us this. Carmella dramatically shows the importance of having others hear and understand us as unique individuals. She needs to be able to think for herself to feel confident about herself, to know who she is, and what she is all about. She needs someone who will encourage and support her thinking to help her develop confidence and self esteem. The need to be heard is basic to our well being, basic to our lives. We all need to be heard.

10. Acknowledge Me

I was working on an acute care inpatient psychiatric unit as a psychiatric nurse. Alicia was twenty-one, in a seclusion room devoid of all furniture, and was running around in the throes of an acute manic psychotic episode. She had just been admitted and put on medication. It would take some time to take effect. She needed a buddy to be with her so she wouldn't hurt herself. The buddy system means that you never leave such a person. As the senior nurse responsible for the nursing care, I had no specific assignments. The staff were very busy, so I said I'd buddy Alicia.

As a former student of Ida Orlando, plus many conversations with her over the years, I am well versed in the importance of never assuming what a patient means. I know how important it is to verify to be sure that what I understand is clearly what that patient means. Also, I know it is important to ascertain whether or not any action I take is or is not helpful. This had been reasonably easy with medical, surgical, and obstetric patients. This had been more difficult with psychiatric patients. But this was my first true test with someone as seriously ill as Alicia with whom I would spend some time. However, I believed we would find a way to communicate and understand each other.

I went into the room and locked myself in with her. Alicia looked at me, then away, and kept running around the room. She was tall and thin. Her tan slacks and matching shirt were clean and wrinkled. Her short hair was tousled and somewhat in her face. She was mumbling, occasionally saying some words, but making no sense. I stated my name, that I was a psychiatric nurse, and that I would buddy her for the next four hours. She didn't look at me. She kept mumbling and running around the room. I gave her space and followed her with my eyes. I acknowledged her by name and told her I would help her in any way I could. She kept running, but gave me a fleeting look. I asked if she'd like to have some ginger ale. No answer. So I waited and stayed quiet. She turned her head quickly toward me, then away, and kept running. "Just let me know in any way you can if I can do anything for you." Alicia gave me another fleeting look and kept running. Sometimes she was nonstop talking, but I still didn't understand a word. I told her I didn't understand, but that I was trying to understand.

I would sometimes get a vague nod. This scenario continued for some time.

Nothing I said seemed to mean anything to her. So I mostly stayed quiet. Then I got a minor nod when I asked, "You must be dry, how about some ginger ale?" Her response gave me some encouragement, so I opened the door, hailed someone outside and asked for some ginger ale. Within five minutes someone handed it to me in a paper cup. I held it out to Alicia. "This is ginger ale. You must be thirsty." She barely slowed down, came close enough to whip it out of my hand and gulp it down. There was more nonstop talking that I didn't understand. I said I'd get some more. I hailed someone again, and was given two more cups full of ginger ale. She drank one, half spilled the other, drank the rest more slowly, then shook her head and put the empty cups into my hand. She was still mostly nonstop talking, and nonstop running. Clearly she was racing and couldn't stay still.

Sometimes when she was talking nonstop she'd look at me as if she wanted me to understand what she was saying. I told her I didn't understand what she was saying, but I would try to understand and I would continue to listen. Sometimes she would spew forth foul language. I had no idea what she meant and didn't feel it was directed at me. I just stayed there quietly, occasionally saying anything that would indicate that I accepted her difficult situation, was trying to understand, and was there to help if I could.

When the four hours were up and another nurse came to buddy her, I said goodbye. I told her I'd see her on the unit when she was better, and that I hoped she'd feel better soon. Another spiel of nonsensical words came forth, including more foul language. So be it. It was a very long four hours and I felt very discouraged. I felt we had not communicated well at all.

Alicia's medication finally took hold and she was let out of the seclusion room. She continued to be full of energy, walked fast around the unit, but would occasionally sit down. She was talkative and lively in her peer group. There was no more foul language and she now made sense. She was very likeable and even tried to help others. However, she was still quite ill and it was decided that she needed longer inpatient care than this short term acute inpatient unit could offer. She was told that she would be transferred to a longer term unit in another hospital. She accepted this more easily than we had expected.

Alicia knew the ambulance would come mid-morning. So, after breakfast she packed with some help, then flew around the unit saying her goodbyes to the staff and patients. After this she hurried over and stopped in front of me. She looked very serious. "I just want to say I'm very sorry I was so mean to you when you were my buddy. I was really nasty to you. I want to apologize. I know you were trying to help me." Her words flew forth in a stream, but were clear. I was astounded and quickly responded. "You don't need to apologize. You were very ill and couldn't help what you were doing." "But I was nasty, I was really nasty. I want you to know I didn't mean it. I really want to apologize." "No apologies necessary," I said. "You were not able to respond in any other way. Your illness was talking, not you."

She continued to look at me with a very serious expression. "You were the only buddy who offered me anything. You were the only buddy who got me some ginger ale. I really appreciated that." A smile flickered across her face as she continued to look at me. I was amazed at what she was saying. She was logical and coherent. She remembered our experience from a few days before, and wanted to share her thoughts and feelings about it. This not only showed some improvement in her illness, she verified that she had understood what had happened and what it meant to her far more than I had realized. She wanted to be sure that I did not misunderstand her or hold any negative feelings about her.

Alicia heard her name called. The ambulance had arrived to take her to the other hospital. She turned toward them to go. As she left she turned back and waved to all of us. Then she looked at me and gave me one final wave with a nod. I waved, smiled, and nodded in return. We heard later that, at her request, the ambulance people let her ride up front with the siren blaring. That was Alicia. She must have had some hell of a ride. We imagined her roaring up the thruway in her glory.

* * *

Mrs. MacGregor, the medication nurse in the acute care unit of a psychiatric hospital, had recently learned the essential features of the Orlando Model. She was doing her best in trying not to make assumptions about whether or not her patients understood what she said or did with them when they did not respond. This afternoon she was giving some medications to two new patients who were mumbling and making no sense. Dillon was twenty-five years old, blond with a small mustache and unkempt beard. He was dressed in a clean light blue rumpled shirt and dungarees. Whitley was thirty-one years old, with brown hair. He had not shaved for a few days. He was dressed in a clean pair of dark green trousers and a rumpled tan shirt. Both had tousled hair. They had been admitted that morning and had settled into the unit. They had eaten lunch, but were unresponsive to anyone who tried to talk with them. The staff had reported that both of them were hearing voices which were not based in reality.

Both patients had come to the medication counter when she motioned to them that it was time for their medication. They were moving about, never keeping still. She turned to one at a time. "Dillon, my name is Mrs. MacGregor. I have some medication for you. It will help you feel better, and help you think more clearly." She gave him the little medication cup with the pills. He took it with a shaking hand, tipped it to his lips, and dropped the pills into his mouth. As he crushed the medication cup in one hand, she put a small cup of water in his outstretched other hand. He took it, drank the water, then gave both cups back to her. Not once did he say anything or make eye contact. He turned and shuffled away.

Whitley had been standing a few feet behind Dillon, patiently waiting his turn. He shuffled over and put out his hand for his medication. "Whitley," she said, "my name is Mrs. MacGregor. This medication will help you feel better, and help you think more clearly." She gave him the medication cup with the pills. Without looking at her, he took the little cup. With his shaking hand he almost spilled the pills on the floor by tipping the cup too soon. Finally he got the tipped cup to his lips, and shook it till the pills dropped into his mouth. He took the little cup and shoved it into his shirt pocket. Then he drank down the water from the next cup she handed him. He still did not look at her. He had been focused on the cups and taking the medication. Without a word he turned and shuffled down the hall.

This similar scenario continued with Mrs. MacGregor, Dillon, and Whitley for the next few days. Then the medication began to take hold. Mrs. MacGregor noticed that Dillon and Whitley had calmed down, were not moving about so much, and seemed more alert. Both had combed hair. Dillon's beard and mustache were clipped and tidy. Whitley had a clean shaven face. Sometimes they were talking together, with other patients, or with staff. It was time for their medication. They saw Mrs. MacGregor at the medication counter and came over without her motioning to them. She looked up to acknowledge them and started to say her name. Dillon immediately held up his hand and interrupted. "I know. You're Mrs. MacGregor. You said this medication will help me think clearly. The voices don't bother me like before." He grinned at her, then took the medication without shaking. He nodded, then turned and left.

Whitley had been distracted by another patient and had not heard Dillon's comments. Mrs. MacGregor realized this, so she started to state her name to him. He, too, stopped her. "I know you're Mrs. MacGregor. You told me this. You told me the medication would help me think better. I am thinking better." He took the medication without shaking. He smiled at her, then turned and wandered off.

In adhering to the Orlando Model, Mrs. MacGregor had been honest with Dillon and Whitley. She knew they understood they were to take the medication, but, because of the severity of their symptoms, she had not believed that either one had understood her name or the reason for the medication. She was still thinking about this and shaking her head in amazement when she told this story to a co-worker as they left the unit at the end of their shift.

* * *

Sam was an outspoken eighty-eight-year-old geriatric hospital patient. Most of his life he had worked as a cobbler in his shoe shop in a small Kentucky town. His diagnosis was progressive dementia. He needed assistance to eat, bathe, and move around his room. He knew who the different people were, but he didn't always know where he was or what year it was. Because of his confusion, his care plan called for frequent reality orientation. One day one of the nurses observed another nurse telling Sam that this was the V.A. Medical Center in Lexington, not Maysville. She emphasized that she wasn't his daughter, she was Pam, a nurse, and she wanted him to open his mouth and eat. Sam not only looked confused. He looked sad. The nurse who saw this realized that the care plan was making him miserable.

A few weeks later Gena, a new volunteer who was not familiar with his care plan, was seen sitting on the bed with Sam kneeling at her feet examining her shoes. He was telling her that she had worn them down at the corner. "If you don't get them fixed, it'll throw your back out. It will, I promise you." She smiled, thanked him, then gently helped him to his feet. After helping him sit down on the bed, she sat beside him. "I'll bet you've fixed lots of shoes, haven't you?" He acknowledged this and beamed. When she left he asked her to stop by the shop tomorrow.

The nurse who observed the difference in Sam between Gena's joining him versus their using reality orientation shared her thoughts about Sam in nursing rounds. She believed they should find out more about his background so they could better join him where he was. Some had doubts, but they agreed to arrange a conference with his daughter. She accepted and eagerly talked about his early days in his shoe shop and the little town in which he'd grown up. She told them about his wife and she showed pictures of Sam in his shop. There he was in his leather apron holding up a shining pair of shoes.

After his daughter left, despite skepticism from some, all agreed to join Sam where he was. If he knew he was in the hospital, he was in the hospital. If he thought he was in his shoe shop, he was in his shoe shop. Soon they noticed a change in Sam. Before this new plan he had been reluctant to attempt his own care. Now, when he believed he had work to do, he'd initiate his own care. He was becoming more independent. They gave him some old shoes which he worked on. He did his own range-of-motion exercises, and his arthritic hands became less stiff. There were less episodes of hostility and he seemed less frustrated.

As Sam's medical condition deteriorated he needed more assistance. Gena, the volunteer, agreed to become Sam's assistant. Over the next few weeks she continued to reassure him that his shoe shop was taken care of, which adequately quelled this periodic concern.

One day Sam told Gena that soon he would be leaving the shop. He wanted to do more fishing. He said he wasn't able to raise her salary, but he'd be happy if she'd be able to do more. She agreed. The day he died he asked his daughter what had she done to this house, that it looked like a hospital. When Gena arrived, he seemed to doze off as he began to detail her assignment for the day. She leaned over and told him she didn't quite understand him. He opened one eye and mumbled, "No more time. I'm goin' fishing." He smiled and closed his eyes for the last time.

The staff grieved over his death. They missed Sam and they missed going to his shop. Some of the nurses went to his funeral. They returned with a gift for the unit from his daughter. She gave them the picture of Sam in his shop that they had seen before. She also gave them a picture of Gena and the nurses in front of Sam's shop. Attached was a note some of which said, "Thank you for allowing Dad to be who he always wanted to be. You gave real meaning to the word 'dignity'." They hung the pictures in the lounge to remind them of their wonderful memories with Sam in Sam's shop.[1]

* * *

Stephen, the physician's assistant (P.A.) assigned to examine five-year-old Sarah, was listening to a brief summary about her from the nurse who had just taken her to an examining room. Sarah had a history of being a very difficult, very uncooperative patient. She had a long medical history with multiple surgeries and frequent trips to her primary care provider. Her blood had been drawn many times. She was terrified of medical personnel, especially if they were wearing white coats. Her mother had brought her to be seen because she had a high fever, and she was very irritable. The nurse's final comment was that Sarah was autistic.

Stephen had never before examined a patient with a diagnosis of autism. He felt some apprehension. At least he could remove his white coat, which he did, leaving it outside the examining room. He walked in. Sarah was sitting on her mother's lap on the examining table. Her cheeks were wet from crying. She was sobbing quietly. He proceeded with his usual procedure with mothers and small children.

He introduced himself. He obtained the essential information about the current situation and relevant medical history by questioning Sarah's mother. Then he stood up in front of both of them. He ignored the fact that Sarah's mother appeared ready to restrain Sarah. He focused on Sarah and explained exactly what he was going to do. He showed her his stethoscope and told her how it worked. He told her about examining her ears and held up the otoscope for her to see.

Sarah reached out for the otoscope and guided Stephen's hand to her ear. Her mother's jaw opened in surprise. Sarah continued to assist Stephen in examining her as he continued to explain what he needed to do. Tears flowed from her mother's eyes. Tears welled up in Stephen's as he continued examining this beautiful little autistic child. Both Sarah's mother and Stephen kept wiping their eyes as Sarah continued to assist with her examination which revealed a severe ear infection. After the examination, the proper medication was dispensed.

Sarah's mother was still in tears as she thanked Stephen as she and her daughter were leaving. She told him she felt that what had happened with their interaction was a significant breakthrough in Sarah's ability to communicate.[2]

* * *

Ida Orlando always believed that people who struggle with psychotic thinking, such as Alicia in the seclusion room, and Dillon and Whitley with the medication nurse, do have some awareness of reality. When we think they are not in reality, part of them does understand some of what is happening. She also believed that even though much of their behavior is determined by their psychotic thinking, some of their behavior does relate to reality. We see this with Alicia when she shows she is able to respond to the offer of ginger ale. We see this with Dillon and Whitley who go to the medication nurse and take their medications. When they are no longer in the throes of their psychotic thinking we learn more. They knew who was with them, and they understood what was happening during those experiences. Alicia is even chagrined about her behavior and feels compelled to apologize. We should never assume that people in these circumstances don't have some awareness of reality. They deserve our honesty, concern, and assistance.

Sam will never recover from his dementia. So it makes sense to go where he is. An elderly friend of our family was in a nursing home because of late life dementia. Like Sam, she had episodic delusional thinking which took her to many far off places. She had traveled to many different countries, so in her way of thinking, she made sense. We all agreed that when we visited with her we would go where ever she was. When we did, those visits were more calm and peaceful than before we realized we should do this.

Autistic children also know more than we may realize. Sarah makes this clear with her responses to Stephen when he joins her in order to have her join him in the examination.

Alicia, Dillon, Whitley, Sam, and Sarah are telling us they are far more aware than we may think. We should not assume otherwise. Each in his or her own way is saying, please do not ignore me, please include me, please acknowledge me.

11. Respect Me

It was a few days after Medical Rounds Review at the Medical Center. That group had deemed Jenny Quinlin's death a suicide from mixing alcohol and sleeping pills. Some from the Psychiatric Department had already believed her death was a suicide. Others in the department said not so fast. They thought the decision was premature. Accidental deaths can occur when alcohol and sleeping pills are combined. So why should suicide be stated as the cause when Medical Rounds Review met only a few days after she was found, and the report from the laboratory that was testing for drugs and alcohol was not yet available. Also, one of the psychiatrists knew other information that had not been included at the review, because a colleague who had been there told him what had been discussed.

No one at the Medical Rounds Review had information from her primary care physician. One physician knew she had been severely depressed, had been seeing a psychiatrist for psychotherapy, and that she had been taking medication for sleep. No one knew what was being addressed in her psychotherapy, nor was there any information about prescriptions. Some believed she had been struggling with an alcohol problem, but no one knew to what degree. Nothing else was presented. After a brief discussion the group agreed that she probably mixed alcohol with whatever she had been taking for sleep, therefore that she had taken her life by suicide.

However, should not more facts have been obtained by the Medical Rounds Review before declaring that Jenny had committed suicide? Professionals who knew either her psychiatrist or her primary care physician decided to combine available information from them with what they heard from people who had worked with her and from people who had known her in the community.

Jenny Quinlin had been retired for many years from a long career as a licensed health care professional at the Medical Center. After her husband died about five years ago, she continued to live in their house by the ocean in an outlying suburb. She rarely came into the city. When she did it was to have lunch or attend events with a friend. Shortly after she lost her husband, she began to have struggles with depression and alcohol. She had thought about suicide, but had always denied that she was actively suicidal. She had never been treated as an inpatient for either a psychiatric or alcohol problem. She was lonely, had been dating an elderly man, but that relationship had dissolved.

She was found dead in her bed one morning by Helena, a neighbor who was a friend. Helena had gone over to see if Jenny would like to go with her to the theater the following month. She knew Jenny would be packing to go to London to visit her daughter, son-in-law, and grandchildren. Jenny had told Helena that she was looking forward to the visit because she hadn't seen them for a year. Helena knew Jenny was very close to her daughter and she missed her, especially after Jenny's husband had died. Helena wanted to see Jenny before she left for the airport.

Jenny was a meticulous person in her actions and in her dress. She was a petite, stunning woman who always looked immaculate at work and in her personal life. Even after she became noticeably depressed she still appeared in clean, well pressed clothes. The evening before the day she was found she had gone out to dinner with a friend. That person said she was quite sure Jenny had only two glasses of wine. She acknowledged that Jenny was somewhat depressed, as she had been for some time, but emphasized that Jenny was looking forward to the London trip. Jenny had looked immaculate, as usual. That was the last time that friend saw her.

The laboratory report finally arrived. Word quickly got around that the report revealed minimal amounts of alcohol and sleeping medication. No other significant information was mentioned. However, the Medical Rounds Review's decision of suicide was not reversed. Those who believed she committed suicide did not change their position. Those who believed her death was accidental were buoyed by adding together all the essential facts.

The laboratory report did not note a high amount of drugs or alcohol. Jenny Quinlin was a retired licensed health care professional who was well acquainted with medications and alcohol problems. Jenny knew the effects of combining alcohol and medications. She had always been a well dressed person even after she became depressed. The evening before she was to pack to go to London on a trip she was looking forward to, she had only two glasses of wine at dinner with a friend.

Is it not possible that she was tired enough to have taken just enough sleeping pills combined with the wine to have accidently pushed herself over the edge? As a petite woman, small amounts of this combination would have affected her more than similar amounts for a larger person. Also, since she was so meticulous about her person and familiar with medications, alcohol, and serious illnesses from her professional work, is it really conceivable that she would have tried to commit suicide with a minimal mix of alcohol and sleeping pills? Would she have wanted to take the chance of not doing the job well enough with the possibility of being left alive with a partially functioning brain or body for all to see?

Those who believed she died accidently emphasized that the combined facts did not warrant the conclusion of suicide. Supported by the compiled information, and out of respect for Jenny, they continued to state that they felt justified in calling her death unfortunate, tragic, and accidental.

* * *

Lili's grandfather, an eighty-six-year-old retired biochemistry professor, lived on an island off the Maine coast. Even though there were great differences in their styles of living, Lili and her family spent many summers with him. She and her husband were orderly early birds. Her grandfather was a sloppy night owl. He never threw anything away. She described how she wanted to clean and empty his house of all sorts of things which to her had no use. But he was a collector. He believed he might need this or that some time now or whenever. She often felt impatient. What she called clutter were items he believed might some day be useful. In hopes of his allowing her to discard some things, she'd get up early and engage him in conversations she believed might make him do what she wanted. The following is one such example.

Knowing he was a nonsmoker, she'd hold up a plastic ashtray she'd found under old tea bags and ask if she could throw it away. He'd reply, "That's for putting your spoon in when you're cooking." She'd return with "But nobody uses it for that." So he'd say, "Give it to me, then. I can keep change in it." He'd take it and pile it on his already cluttered desk. She would find her voice rising as she'd finally retort with "But you can't keep everything.

There's so much stuff, you can't buy new things." His response was immediate. "Exactly," he'd say. End of that round.

As the summers went on she'd realize more and more that his way of living held much meaning for him. She became aware that she too easily failed to fully appreciate how her grandfather's memories of her late grandmother were involved in that Maine house. For example, she was eager to discard her grandmother's mildewed, yellow rain hat. He, of course, wanted to keep it. She realized she had been struggling with living with his ways, yet he accepted their ways, including those of her young daughter, Madeline. He didn't mind Madeline's strewn toys and crusty Play-Doh. Madeline and her "Super Grampy" even had some things in common. Both wore bibs, napped in the afternoon, and insisted on ice cream for desert.

Lili was aware that many of her friends barely got through holiday weekends with their relatives without losing patience. It occurred to her that when she didn't take the time to understand her grandfather, she missed what he had to offer. When she began to appreciate what his ways meant to him, and how much she recognized what she was learning from him, she viewed him differently. By then she was pleased to realize she could give him the respect he deserved.[1]

* * *

Christie already knew she would be judged by her occupation. In social situations with people she didn't know, they would acknowledge her name, then ask, "And what do you do?" When she replied that she was a reporter they usually responded with some deference. When she was at her job, strangers were generally courteous and friendly. People sounded respectful when they telephoned. Then she decided to leave her reporter's job to wait on tables while figuring out what she wanted to do next.

As a waitress Christie found herself being treated in a wide variety of ways by her customers.

She would introduce herself with "Hi, my name is Christie," then wait for eye contact. Sometimes she'd stand quietly for an awkwardly long time waiting for a response. She admitted she was trying to convey that she was a person, too, and that she wanted some respect.

When she had waited tables during summers, she felt that many people treated her like a peon until she told them she was in college. This time she had no recourse. Some would stare at the menu and mumble drink orders while refusing to look at her. Some would interrupt her to say that the air conditioner was too cold or that the sun was too bright as it came through the windows. One evening a man waved her away when he was on his cell phone. A minute or so later he beckoned her with his finger and complained that he wondered where she had been because he was ready to order.

Christie often saw co-workers storm into the kitchen in tears or swearing because a customer had interrupted, degraded, or ignored them. Almost daily she heard them mutter in various ways that people shouldn't be treated like that.

After eight months she left the restaurant to take an office job. She found some civility in the relationships there. She decided to apply to graduate school and go on to a profession. Even then, she thought, if people want something from me, they'll have to be nice to me. Maybe I'll take them to dinner to see how they treat someone whose only job is to serve them.[2]

* * *

Tom didn't realize he was a nerd until he began school. His enthusiasm for answering teachers' questions made some of his classmates think he was deliberately trying to make them look bad. Bullies went after him on the playground. He managed to hold his ground because he was tall. He survived in class by keeping quiet.

Later he became a high school teacher because he believed there were many young nerds who needed to know how wonderful it is to be a nerd. Each year he invited his Advanced Placement physics students to his house for study sessions before the Advanced Placement test. One year a mother of one of those students told Tom that her son had returned home after one of those sessions and talked for hours about how awesome it was to have found a nerd family.

Then he raised two nerd sons. His daughter described herself as a nerd sympathizer. His sons were picked on by classmates. His older son was an easy target because he was pale and not athletic. Bullies harassed him every afternoon while he waited for the school bus. They derided him for his brilliance such as when he cited the periodic table of elements from memory when the teacher only asked for anyone to name any element. He went to karate class, was given pep talks by his parents, but was never able to win the respect of those who tormented him.

Both sons were misunderstood by their teachers. His younger son's middle school social studies teacher insisted he take notes. He refused. So in front of the class she told him he'd never graduate from high school. To his Dad he insisted it was illogical to write notes because he remembered what she said, and doing so cut into his thinking time. So he and his Dad discussed options. They finally agreed that he could write the notes backward. This was easy because, as a child, he used to entertain his parents by turning books upside down and reading them backward. Problem solved. His teacher never noticed.

His older son hitchhiked around Europe three times and learned to speak four foreign languages. Though he remained a nerd, by then he was not considered a sissy. A group of Russian policemen gave him a party after he accepted their invitation for a December dip in a spring of near-freezing water.

His younger son proved his teacher wrong by graduating from high school. He scored the top score on the Scholastic Aptitude Test and was asked to give a speech before 500 educators and politicians. They had gathered to honor education. Tom could not stop worrying about how his son would manage this commitment. He had no idea what he would say.

His son got up from his seat. All eyes were on him. He went, stood where expected, and looked out at the now quiet audience. Then he delivered ten minutes of stand-up comedy about being a nerd. The audience was spellbound. They laughed until they cried. Tom could not stop his tears. After this superb performance Tom's son received his highest compliment from a young nerd. "Thank you for what you've done for our people."

For both sons, respect at last.[3]

* * *

No matter how old we are we want to be treated with respect. We want others to respect us when they refer to us or take any action that affects us.

The combined information about Jenny Quinlin and her death was stronger in support of ruling her death an accident rather than an act of suicide. Despite that, the initial official conclusion of suicide based on incomplete information was not changed. Even if the combined information had been equivocal, shouldn't that have been so stated? Suicides can leave deep hurt and sometimes guilt in families and close friends who feel that maybe they should have seen this coming, maybe they should have been aware enough to have prevented it. If the evidence is not strong enough to support suicide, why tell people it was and leave them struggling with such thoughts and feelings? Shouldn't we respect the person and those near them by calling it what it more likely was, an accident, or if we don't know, that it could well have been an accident? Isn't that more reasonable?

Lili's struggles with her grandfather's ways which were so different from her own is a familiar scenario. It can be difficult when people with different styles of living share the same living space. Ideally they begin to learn from each other as well as finding ways to accommodate to each other without expecting either to make unwanted sacrifices. Ultimately Lili realizes that her grandfather has accepted what he hasn't been used to, such as her daughter's strewn toys, and she comes to respect how much many things in his Maine house remind him of his past with her deceased grandmother. Taking the time to listen and to understand, she finally begins to learn from him and to respect him.

People such as Christie whose work involves giving service to others are sometimes treated poorly. Persons who behave as if those in service occupations are beneath them may or may not even think about what they are doing. Maybe something in their lives will eventually occur which will result in their being aware of such attitudes and, concomitantly, result in a change in their behavior.

Tom and his sons should remind us that we too often view others through stereotypical thinking. Whether we are teachers, peers, or whoever we are, if we take the time, we can get to know others as unique individuals and come to respect them.

If we are not aware of our assumptions, they can mislead. In listening to understand, we can better appreciate an essential human need: that we all feel the need to have others respect us.

12. Our Doctors Need Our Stories

All health professionals who make diagnostic and treatment decisions (e.g. physicians, nurse practitioners, physician assistants, various mental health practitioners) must develop the ability to listen and ascertain the essential information needed from a patient's story. Professionals responsible for triage decisions, immediately ascertaining whether a situation is urgent or not, also need patients' stories for their decisions. Any patient's story may need to include facts available from other relevant persons. Patients' stories are important for patient care decisions as well as triage, diagnostic, and treatment decisions. The sometimes complex issues involved in making diagnostic and treatment decisions are usually the responsibility of our physicians.

Our doctors need to acknowledge us, respect us, and listen to us, because they need to understand us and accurately diagnose and treat us. Despite their training and experience, or sometimes because of it, they have their own assumptions and biases.

For a number of years Lisa Sanders, M.D., has been writing the column "Diagnosis" for *The New York Times Magazine*. Her stories present complex medical situations with puzzling diagnoses. As in her book, *Every Patient Tells a Story*, she notes that the patient's story is not only the oldest diagnostic tool, it is often the best place to find the clue that unravels the mystery. Even with modern technology, 70% to 90% of diagnoses are based on the patient's story alone.[1]

Sir William Osler, M.D., the father of modern medicine, told his medical students that "the best teaching is that taught by the patient himself."[2] Some time ago I accompanied my brother-in-law to our hospital emergency service. Though he had been through triage, the doctor said to him, "Talk to me as if I know nothing about you. Tell me your story from the beginning." This was music to my ears, as it is with any of my doctors when they request the same from me.

*　*　*

Nathan was a hefty 140 pound, four-foot-eight-inch fourth grade Hopi Indian boy who attended his local Hopi school in rural Arizona. He reveled in rough and tumble play. Just at the end of school recess another student jumped on his back for a piggyback ride. Nathan immediately fell to the ground screaming in pain. He was terrified, sobbing and moaning as he was brought into the emergency department on a backboard which immobilized his spine.

Dr. Harrison Alter, the physician who listened to his story, found that Nathan could move his arms and legs. There was no tingling nor did Nathan have the feeling of electric shocks going down his spine, but he complained of terrible pain in the middle of his back. The X-ray showed a compression fracture of the tenth thoracic vertebra. The tests for a complete blood count, calcium level, and bone enzymes were normal. The computed tomography (CT) scan, transmitted digitally to a radiologist at the University of Arizona, and magnetic resonance imaging (MRI) for which Nathan had to travel to Flagstaff, an hour and a half away, all showed the collapsed vertebra, no other abnormalities. Dr. Alter obtained these latter tests because Nathan's story and medical results didn't make sense. He did not understand why a compression fracture from a piggyback ride in an overweight but otherwise healthy ten-year-old Hopi boy should have occurred. Dr. Alter was puzzled because this type of fracture was what he more often saw in eighty-year-old women.

So Dr. Alter called a local pediatrician. "We just see this sometimes," said the specialist, who told Dr. Alter that he and the family should not worry. Dr. Alter felt he could do no more, but he could not get Nathan out of his mind.

Some weeks later Nathan got out of bed and immediately collapsed in pain. The X-rays taken after he returned to the emergency department showed four wedge fractures in his spine. Dr. Alter transferred Nathan to a Phoenix hospital where a bone biopsy performed by an orthopedic surgeon was sent to a Phoenix pathologist. Special tests done on abnormal cells found inside the bone finally led to the diagnosis. Nathan had acute lymphoblastic leukemia. The leukemia had weakened the vertebrae which had collapsed when the other boy jumped on Nathan for the piggyback ride. Puzzle solved.

Dr. Alter had believed that Nathan's story that brought him to the emergency department with the first fracture had not made sense. His final comment from this situation was that no one, either physician or patient, should ever accept "we see this sometimes" as a first answer to a serious event. It is important to keep looking until what is wrong has been identified and resolved.[3]

* * *

Dr. Jerome Groopman tells of an elderly man who came to the emergency room complaining of ankle pain after tripping on the street. All he wanted was something for the pain and reassurance that his ankle wasn't fractured. Since that is what he presented, that is what the physician and staff focused on. Only later did they learn that he had fallen because he was weak from undiagnosed anemia caused by colon cancer. No one thought to ask why he had tripped.[4]

* * *

Dr. Myron Falchuk, a gastroenterologist, described his patient, Joe Stern, as a "wonderful, delightful character from the old country." Joe, in his late eighties, was still spry, drove around the city, and took adult education classes. Joe's chief complaint was indigestion which he described as heartburn. General practitioners and internists usually treat such patients. However, Dr. Falchuk knew the Sterns, so he accepted Joe as his patient. Dr. Falchuk so enjoyed Joe Stern's company that he let him stay over the allotted time for each visit. They kibitzed together in Yiddish, and Dr. Falchuk admitted he also enjoyed Joe's great sense of humor.

Joe's indigestion went on for several weeks. Dr. Falchuk treated him with antacids and various medications. Despite only slight relief over four months, Dr. Falchuk kept adjusting Joe's medications. He was aware he just didn't want to put Joe through invasive tests. Then Joe arrived feeling faint and exhausted. This was different. Joe had become anemic. So Dr. Falchuk followed through by doing an upper endoscopy which involved snaking a fiberoptic instrument down Joe's throat into his esophagus and stomach. Large growths were present. A biopsy confirmed that cancer that had been there all the time accounted for his persistent indigestion.

Fortunately the cancer was treatable, the delay in diagnosis didn't harm Joe, and he went into remission. However, Dr. Falchuk admitted that he missed the diagnosis because he didn't want to subject this delightful, elderly man to the discomfort and strain of the endoscopy procedure.[5]

* * *

As chief of Infectious Disease at a renowned hospital, Dr. Tony Biondi was experienced and very knowledgeable about a wide variety of illnesses caused by bacteria, viruses, protozoa, fungi, and "everything else in any way related to a microbe." His most memorable patient was Harold Bernstein, a forty-five-year-old electronics engineer with a disease whose clinical characteristics resembled aseptic meningitis, an inflammation of the tissues surrounding the spinal cord. Harold had the usual symptoms of fever, headache, and stiff neck. However, a tap of his spinal fluid told Dr. Biondi to look for some other, less common cause of Harold's symptoms.

Numerous complex physiological and tissue studies were done. Various consultants were called in including some from all sections of the Department of Internal Medicine. Dr. Biondi spent innumerable hours reviewing the literature and contacting colleagues all over the world. He even consulted surgeons. Despite all these efforts Harold Bernstein's condition became progressively worse. He developed many debilitating symptoms and moved closer and closer to death.

Dr. Biondi tried one antibiotic, then another. He tried other pharmacological agents. No effect. No change. Dr. Biondi visited Harold daily, more often as his health continued to deteriorate. Dr. Biondi knew that Harold was an engineer married to an architect, and that he was used to dealing with very specific information. So, from the beginning Dr. Biondi was specific when he shared information, hiding nothing from either Harold or his wife, Etta. Every time he visited Harold, he admitted to both of them that he was no closer to a diagnosis than when Harold was initially evaluated. Time and time again Dr. Biondi told them that he and his colleagues didn't really know what they were doing. But Harold and Etta also knew Dr. Biondi was continuing to pursue anything that might result in a diagnosis and anything that might make Harold better. His efforts and the honest and trusting relationship Harold and Etta had with him continued to give them hope.

Because of that reliable relationship, combined with the enormous effort Dr. Biondi was making to find an accurate diagnosis and workable treatment plan, Harold and Etta never lost confidence in their dedicated physician. "Confidence" was their word, said Dr. Biondi when he related this story. They told him they had confidence in him almost every time they talked with him.

Somewhere around the third week of hospitalization Harold was no longer getting worse. For a few days his condition remained unchanged. Then he slowly began to get better. His continual improvement amazed Dr. Biondi and the many involved professionals. They had never seen such a remarkable course of recovery. Before the end of two more weeks Harold was well enough to be discharged home where he continued to improve. When Dr. Biondi made home visits, he and the Bernsteins shared their memories of what they had been through. On each of those visits the Bernsteins mentioned to Dr. Biondi what they had always said, that they never lost confidence in him. Harold believed that his confidence in his dedicated physician was responsible for the good outcome. Even five years later there was no recurrence.[6]

* * *

The first in a series of reports from the Quality of Health Care in America project was published in 2000. This project was initiated by the Institute of Medicine (IOM) in 1998. This first report, *To Err Is Human: Building a Safer Health System,* is concerned with patient safety. The report notes that more people in United States hospitals die in a given year as a result of medical errors than from motor vehicle accidents, breast cancer, or AIDS.[7]

Lisa Sanders, M.D., in her book, *Every Patient Tells a Story,* notes that a researcher who searched the text of that famous IOM report noted that the term "medication error" came up seventy times, but the term "diagnostic error" occurred only twice. She believes that even though the IOM report noted that diagnostic errors accounted for 17% of all the errors made, research into the cause and solution of diagnostic errors is in its infancy. Studies suggest that 10% to 15% of primary care patients (those seen in internal medicine, family medicine, and pediatrics) are given an incorrect diagnosis. Diagnostic errors may have no effect if the patients get better without further care or if they return when their symptoms become worse. But diagnostic errors that hurt patients or lead to deaths are a major concern.[8]

In his book *How Doctors Think*, Jerome Groopman, M.D., also notes the lack of discussion about misdiagnosis in the IOM report. Misdiagnosis involves looking into the thinking process involved in making a diagnosis. He notes that experts who studied this issue concluded that the majority of diagnostic errors are due to flaws in physician thinking, not due to technical mistakes. One of those flaws is that physicians fail to question their assumptions.[9] Dr. Sanders also believes that the most common diagnostic errors involve how doctors think. She believes the most common diagnostic error is premature closure.[10]

Both these doctors want physicians to think creatively and not dismiss data that doesn't fit, to keep searching for a diagnosis if a patient isn't getting better, and to ask what else could this be rather than latching onto the first possible diagnosis.[11] In other words the story should include all needed information, should not have pieces that don't fit, and any assumptions made should be verified to ascertain whether or not they are correct.

In the first story in Chapter 1, Dr. McKay didn't go to Mavis' hospital room to ask her why she pulled the fire alarm. Instead he called me from the mental health service with the urgent request that I transfer her to the state psychiatric hospital. Dr. McKay assumed that Mavis was still struggling with psychotic thinking that had led to his admitting her for a medication change. He believed she was still hearing voices and that her thoughts were still confused. Had he gone to her room and asked her why she pulled the alarm and asked if she were still hearing voices, he would have realized she was better. "Pull a fire alarm if you can't find a policeman or fireman, and someone will come and help you," Mavis told me. She said she had learned this from her mother when she was a child. When the nurse ushered her back to her room and turned up the lights, Mavis immediately knew where she was. She knew the medication had cleared her thinking. Both Dr. McKay and the nurse believed the previous information, not the present information so readily available had either of them just talked with her.

"Verify, verify," said Orlando to her students and colleagues. "Assumptions may be correct or incorrect. You just don't know until you get verification," she would state with emphasis.

Dr. Harrison Alter wants us to remember that treatment and resolution of a patient's medical situation must be considered in combination with the patient's story. There should be no lingering puzzles. Information from the story, diagnosis, treatment, and outcome must be considered as a whole in order to ascertain if the outcome is reasonable. Dr. Alter recognized that Nathan's fracture from the attempted piggyback ride didn't make sense in a presumably healthy ten-year-old boy who reveled in rough and tumble play. He obtained a CT scan and an MRI. But the puzzle remained. Premature closure. The final diagnosis became clear when more fractures ensued and more tests were done. Dr. Alter has already reminded us never to accept "we see this sometimes" as a final answer to a serious puzzling event that has not yet been adequately solved.

As for the elderly man who fell and wanted to know if he had fractured his ankle, this was premature closure at its best. The physician and staff incorrectly assumed that the presenting symptom in this patient's story was all they needed to adequately treat him. It appears they were viewing him through the bias of stereotypical thinking. Elderly folks can fall and fracture their bones. But elderly or otherwise, we are all unique. This man who fell deserved a full assessment to include information about his current health, whether or not falls were usual for him, and the circumstance in which he fell. Encouraging him to complete his story, or obtaining it from others if needed, might have led them to a more thorough assessment which might have revealed the underlying medical problems: his anemia and his cancer.

Dr. Falchuk liked Joe Stern so much, he just didn't want him to suffer through an invasive endoscopy procedure. Even though Joe's situation didn't appreciably change, Dr. Falchuk believed it was reasonable to continue to treat him with antacids and various medications. Another assumption not verified. There was more to Joe's symptoms than Dr. Falchuk had allowed himself to believe. A comfortable, even likeable, relationship between doctors and their patients can promote good care. However, in such a relationship our doctors may avoid procedures they know will be arduous for us. That avoidance can prevent thoroughness and may be detrimental in giving us quality care. If a medical situation doesn't improve, there is more to consider.

Dr. Toni Biondi put his knowledge, experience, heart, and soul into ascertaining the cause of Harold's severe illness and in finding a viable treatment plan. He never wavered in his attempts to save this forty-five-year-old man from what all the professionals had begun to think would be inevitable death. No diagnosis was found and no treatment worked. But here we have a dedicated physician who sought all possible tests and consultations to find a reason for Harold's worsening condition. He never ceased in his quest to find a diagnosis and to find a cure. His efforts and trusting relationship with Harold and Etta gave them confidence and gave them hope. Harold always believed that his confidence in his dedicated physician is what pulled him through.

Our doctors need our stories as a starting point to think through a reasonable diagnosis and treatment plan. In doing so they need to recognize and verify any assumptions. Our stories can also help them better understand us and contribute to fostering a relationship that can be crucial in giving us confidence and hope, sometimes the most critical ingredients for a cure.

13. How We Hear Our Doctors

The Hurlburts lived in Buffalo, New York, when their son was born with congenital hydrocephalus (excess accumulation of cerebrospinal fluid in the brain). The usual treatment is a permanent shunt to drain the excess fluid to the abdomen. Excess fluid enlarges the skull, which can easily be ascertained by measuring the person's head with a tape measure. Since his birth he had been followed in Buffalo by a professor of neurosurgery.

The Hurlburt's son was four years old when the family moved to a small town in rural Vermont where the local pediatrician began to follow him. Mrs. Hurlburt had been told by the professor in Buffalo that the hydrocephalus was arrested, therefore no shunt was required. She understood that the professor had wanted to see her son every three months so his head could be measured and questions could be asked about his development. The pediatrician guessed that the frequent visits may have been scheduled to reassure her. Her behavior indicated otherwise. He found himself in the presence of an extremely anxious mother.

At their first visit her son appeared normal except that his head was minimally increased in size. The pediatrician was not worried about him. He was worried about his mother. Mrs. Hurlburt was intensely anxious that her son's hydrocephalus might be insidiously progressing and causing brain damage. She had not been comfortable with the professor's care. She could not understand why he had evaluated him with a simple tape measure. She had expected other tests and surgery. She believed she needed to watch her son every second lest she miss something terrible that might happen. She told the pediatrician that when she was in Buffalo the professor referred her to a psychiatrist for her anxiety. She had not accepted his reassurances, so he put her on a tranquilizer, which she was still taking.

The pediatrician realized he needed to spend more time with Mrs Hurlburt to better understand her thinking. He decided to listen to her story. In a lengthy conversation she revealed the rationale underlying her concerns. She could not understand why her son was being seen every three months if his hydrocephalus were arrested. If her son's situation were truly arrested, then why the frequent visits. It made no sense to her unless the professor thought something else might reveal itself.

Because Mrs. Hurlburt's son's head size was only slightly increased, the pediatrician decided not to see him every three months. He would measure the boy's head only at his regular check-ups. He believed too much attention had been paid to this little boy. However, he felt he should share his new treatment plan with the Buffalo professor. He found out that the professor had retired, so he talked by phone with the new chief of neurosurgery. That chief was reluctant to change the former chief's plan, but finally agreed to support the revised plan.

The pediatrician regularly saw this boy for another five years before leaving to join a group in Boston, Massachusetts. He measured the boy's head only on every other visit. Mrs. Hurlburt stopped taking her tranquilizer. On her son's twenty-first birthday she wrote to this conscientious pediatrician in Boston and told him that no one had measured her son's head in years. She wrote that her son was fine and a junior at the University of Vermont.[1]

* * *

Dr. Bernard Lown witnessed the following situation during his training in cardiology with Dr. Samuel Levine at the Peter Bent Brigham Hospital, Boston, Massachusetts. Dr. Levine made patient rounds once a week with his entourage of trainees. He would quickly examine and ask questions of each patient, dialogue with his trainees, say a few encouraging words to the patient, then move on. When he talked with either his trainees or patients, he expected succinct responses. Though revealing important information, each cursory visit rarely lasted more than five minutes.

One patient in her early forties had been a clinic patient for more than thirty years. She revered Dr. Levine who had treated her since childhood when rheumatic fever had left her with a severely scarred and narrowed tricuspid heart valve. Severe bloating from excess fluid in her legs and abdomen were her constant symptoms. Despite the struggle she continued her work as a librarian. Dr. Lown heard Dr. Levine mutter that she was a decent and brave woman, which indicated that the admiration went both ways.

On this particular morning she was experiencing much congestion that had not responded to treatment. When she saw

Dr. Levine she was optimistic with the expectation that he would solve this problem because he had solved her medical problems on many previous occasions. However, he was more hurried than usual. Visitors were overwhelming him, many physicians were crowding close to hear his latest pearls, and he was perfunctory when he briefly examined her.

Dr. Levine barked out to his trainees that this was a case of TS, medical jargon for tricuspid stenosis. He moved on while Dr. Lown and some other trainees remained to listen to this woman's heart. Usually this stoic woman was quiet. This time she became increasingly anxious and agitated. To the trainees, now alone with her, she murmured "This is the end." Dr. Lown asked her why she was so upset. She answered that Dr. Levine said she had TS. She began to cry. He asked her what she thought it meant. Through her tears she replied. "It means terminal situation."

Dr. Lown knew her interpretation was incorrect. Patients with tricuspid stenosis may waste away and slowly die. But her heart did not have a diseased and failing left ventricle which results in congestion different from her congestion. He attempted to explain and reassure her. She heard nothing of what he said. Her breathing became rapid and labored. For the first time she could not lie back. Her struggle to breathe forced her to sit bolt upright.

Dr. Lown reexamined her. Her lungs had been completely clear. Now she showed severe lung congestion. A chest X-ray confirmed that her lungs were flooded with fluid. She was immediately admitted to a medical ward where neither oxygen, morphine, nor diuretics to flush out the excess fluid made any difference.

Dr. Lown called Dr. Levine and told him about these startling events. Dr. Levine replied that people with tricuspid stenosis don't behave this way clinically. His voice seem to imply that he doubted what he was hearing. He promised he would see this woman that evening after making rounds on his private patients. Her lungs became progressively overwhelmed. She died before Dr. Levine arrived. Dr. Lown "stood transfixed, helpless and aghast" as he witnessed this final scenario.[2]

* * *

As a cardiologist some years later, Dr. Lown was responsible for a sixty-year-old man who was in coronary intensive care because of many complications after a severe heart attack. Nearly all his heart muscle had been destroyed. He was in congestive heart failure, and all possible treatments had not improved his condition. He was weak and had no energy to eat. His sleep was disrupted from difficulty breathing and lack of oxygen. He was pasty looking, and he periodically gasped for air as if he were drowning.

Each morning on rounds Dr. Lown and his staff entered his room looking more as if they were undertakers than physicians. They believed they had nothing else to offer. They chose not to reassure him because they felt that would insult his intelligence and undermine his trust in them. They hurried their visits so as not to face his questioning stare any longer than necessary. The situation deteriorated each day. After consulting with the patient's family, Dr. Lown pulled out his chart and wrote "do not resuscitate."

Then one morning Dr. Lown noticed that this patient's vital signs had improved. This severely ill man looked better and said he felt better. Dr. Lown still did not think he would survive, but did believe that a change in environment might be less stressful. He transferred him to a less intensive care unit where he lost track of him.

Six months later this patient was back at Dr. Lown's office. Though his heart was severely damaged, there was no congestion. Dr. Lown was incredulous and exclaimed that his improvement must be some miracle.

"No miracle . . . I know the exact moment when this so called miracle happened," he said without hesitating. He explained that he knew that Dr. Lown and his staff were at their wits end and didn't know what to do. Because of their behavior he, too, thought he was dying.

Then, "on Thursday morning, April twenty-fifth, you came in with your gang, surrounded the bed, and looked as though I was already in a casket. You put your stethoscope on my chest and urged everyone to listen to the wholesome gallop." He went on to explain that he understood this to mean that his heart was still capable of a healthy gallop, therefore he couldn't really be dying. He never knew nor was he ever told that a gallop was a bad sign, that it was a sound caused by an overstretched failing left ventricle straining ineffectively to pump blood.[3]

* * *

Bernie Siegel, M.D., writes about a woman diagnosed with a malignant brain tumor. She was given three months to live. She was desperate, so she went to Mexico for laetrile treatment. A year later she felt well, and she was doing well. She was driving her car, and she had returned to work.

Then she unexpectedly came upon the doctor she had originally seen. He expressed shock and surprise to see that she was still living. So she told him about her laetrile treatment in Mexico. He was indignant. He emphasized that laetrile treatment was quackery, and berated her for wasting her time and money. He said he could show her proof about what he was saying. Responding to his pronouncements, she died that night.[4]

* * *

Mr. Wright was severely ill with advanced lymphosarcoma, a malignancy that involved his lymph nodes. Huge tumors the size of oranges were in his neck, armpits, groin, chest, and abdomen. His spleen and liver were enormous. His thoracic duct was obstructed. One to two liters of milky fluid was drawn from his chest every other day. He frequently required oxygen. Because no further treatments were considered viable, none were scheduled. Sedatives were given to ease his pain. Mr. Wright was considered terminal.

Then he heard that the clinic where he was a patient was one of a hundred selected to evaluate Krebiozen, a new drug which might help his condition. But Mr. Wright was ineligible because the twelve patients accepted for this trial had to have a life expectancy of at least three or preferably six months. To suggest that Mr. Wright might last more than two weeks was absurd. He was not considered for the trial.

A few days later the new drug arrived. Mr. Wright refused to accept that he had been excluded from receiving it. He begged his physician, Dr. West, to give him this new drug which he believed was his "golden opportunity." Mr. Wright begged so vigorously that, against the rules of the Krebiozen committee and against his own better judgment, Dr. West relented and included him as one of the twelve who would receive the drug.

Injections were scheduled for three times a week. Mr. Wright received his first Krebiozen injection on Friday. That day Dr. West noted that Mr. Wright had a fever, was gasping for air, and was completely bedridden. Given how moribund Mr.Wright was that Friday, when Dr. West returned on Monday he thought Mr. Wright might be dead and his injections could go to another patient more suitable for the trial. Dr. West was incredulous when he found Mr. Wright walking around chatting happily with the nurses, spreading good cheer to anyone who would listen. His tumors had decreased to half their original size, impossible from any treatment that might have otherwise been suitable. Dr. West quickly evaluated the other patients in the trial. They showed either no change or a change for the worse.

The schedule was continued, and Mr. Wright was given the Krebiozen injections three times a week. Within ten days he was discharged. By then he was breathing normally and was fully active including flying in his plane. Dr. West remained astounded.

Within two months conflicting reports about the efficacy of Krebiozen appeared in the news. All the clinics that were testing this drug reported no results. The originators of the treatment still believed in their new drug and attempted to contradict the discouraging news. As the weeks went on Mr. Wright became considerably disturbed by the disappointing information. He began to lose faith in what he considered was his last hope. As the reports became increasingly dismal, he became extremely discouraged and, after two months of nearly perfect health, he relapsed to his earlier severe medical condition.

Because Dr. West was so impressed with Mr. Wright's stunning improvement from the first injections, he decided to be less than truthful with him. He told Mr. Wright he should not believe the newspapers, that Krebiozen was a promising drug. Mr. Wright countered by asking Dr. West why he had relapsed. Dr. West told him Krebiozen deteriorates on standing. A new super-refined, double-strength Krebiozen was to arrive soon which would more than reproduce the results of the original drug. Mr. Wright looked interested.

Dr. West delayed a few days until Mr. Wright's enthusiasm and faith reached a peak, then offered him a double-strength dose of a fresh preparation of the newly arrived Krebiozen. Mr. Wright was ecstatic. With much fanfare Dr. West injected him with sterile water. Mr. Wright recovered from this second near terminal state even more dramatically than before. His tumors melted, his chest fluid disappeared, he walked and even returned to flying. He appeared the picture of good health. Because of Mr. Wright's faith in this new treatment, Dr. West continued the sterile water injections. For the next two months Mr. Wright was without his symptoms.

Then a final American Medical Association announcement appeared in the press: "nationwide tests show Krebiozen to be a worthless drug in the treatment of cancer." Within a few days of this report Mr. Wright was readmitted to the hospital with full exacerbation of his severe medical condition. He died less than two days later.[5]

* * *

Dr. Bernard Lown remembers Tony, a handsome elderly Italian with stunning white hair, who was dying from end stage cardiomyopathy, a severe heart muscle disease. Tony was mostly silent. If he spoke, it would be in brief, one syllable words. Only the subject of his pigeons, which he bred, raced, and loved, would rouse him. His drooping eyelids and brooding manner were ever present. He could not be cheered. His constant companion was Lisa, a beautiful young woman who responded to his every need. Dr. Lown told Tony he was lucky to have such a devoted daughter. Tony corrected him. "Doc, she's my mistress." So a few days later Dr Lown said in a somewhat teasing manner, "You should marry her." Tony's immediate reply was that he didn't want to leave a widow immediately after a wedding. "Who says you will?" responded his devoted doctor.

Tony told Dr. Lown that he'd make a deal with him. He said Lisa was eager to marry. He told his doctor that if he would guarantee in writing that he'd be around for five years, he'd follow his advice. So Dr Lown drafted a statement guaranteeing without equivocation that Tony would live five years. Tony improved and was soon discharged from the hospital. A few days later Dr. Lown received a post card from the honeymooning couple. Though appreciated, this did not reassure Dr. Lown who frequently worried about having impulsively written and given Tony this questionable statement.

Five years later Tony returned looking none the worse for the five years. Lisa looked more beautiful than ever and was deeply in love. "The five years are up, Doc. I need a new contract," stated Tony. So Dr. Lown responded by once again writing the same type of contract.

Another five years passed. Tony returned. Though calm and carrying himself with dignity, he was struggling to breathe, his body was weighed down with edema, and his abdomen was hugely distended. He was severely ill and feeling miserable. He did not request another contract. Dr. Lown admitted him to the hospital and treated him for his symptoms, making him as comfortable as possible. Despite his grave condition, Tony lived two more years.[6]

* * *

Joe Dennet was a renowned director of Canterbury's rare book library. As a knowledgeable curator, his persistent and shrewd negotiations had resulted in major bequests of money, manuscripts, and books to the library. Stories about his acquisitions of many of those treasures were legendary. He had not only tracked down rare valuable books from a wide range of people, such as the likes of the Vanderbilts to various questionable characters, he kept scrupulous records on every transaction. Many of Joe's own stories included much that was not recorded. His vast knowledge about his work included intimate impressions of all sorts of book people, as well as intricate details of some of his most intriguing negotiations.

Dr. Louis Kronberg, his cardiologist, also interested in rare books and their early history, was fascinated with Joe's stories. He first began to take care of Joe when Joe was admitted to the emergency room with a major heart attack when he was fifty-seven. This was followed by a series of complications which ultimately required urgent coronary artery bypass surgery. Then Joe did well for many years. During those years Joe and Dr. Kronberg shared their interest in rare books in conversations when Joe saw him as a patient and at the library which Dr. Kronberg visited a few times each year.

Joe worked every day at the library until the mandatory retirement age of seventy. Then he was given a small office in the library which allowed him to continue to work as much as he wished. About a year later he had another severe heart attack which resulted in worsening congestive heart failure over the next four years. His heart could not maintain a beat of its own, so a defibrillator was implanted. Dr. Kronberg and his colleagues were not able to control his downhill course. Joe was no longer able to go to his beloved library. Increasingly he struggled with emotional anguish. Since this remarkable man had long been as much a friend as a patient, Dr. Kronberg shared his emotional pain. He began to see Joe weekly instead of monthly and kept trying to figure out some way to revive his spirits.

At the end of one of Joe's visits, Joe watched Dr. Kronberg carefully write out a prescription. Joe was surprised because it had been a long time since he had been given any prescriptions. His eyes brightened as he looked at it. The prescription showed only four words: "One set of memoirs." Joe lingered at these words. Then his face lit up with a smile that Dr. Kronberg hadn't seen in weeks. As Joe left the office he looked at the doctor he so revered and cheerfully said, "I've told you a few of these stories, but even you will be surprised at what's in this book, I promise you."

Within days, daily for hours at a time, he dictated to his daughter-in-law. She was so pleased with the change in him that she devoted any time he wanted to work with her. Though he was limited by his cardiac insufficiency and breathing difficulties, the project progressed more quickly than Dr. Kronberg had hoped. Joe's medical condition didn't improve, but Joe seemed like a different man as he told Dr. Kronberg about the book's progress at his outpatient visits.

A little more than three months after acknowledging the prescription, Joe's wife brought him in for his weekly appointment in his wheelchair. He could not complete a sentence without stopping several times to breathe, but he looked up with what Dr. Kronberg said could only be an expression of triumph. A photocopy of the manuscript of his completed memoirs was tucked under his arm. He had dedicated it to Dr. Kronberg. A copy of the prescription was centered on page one.

Joe was now ready to die. Neither Joe nor Dr. Kronberg wanted him to die from drowning as his lungs filled with fluid, which would be the result of congestive heart failure. At his next office visit they agreed to have his defibrillator turned off. At home, three days later, two hours before his defibrillator was to be turned off, he died suddenly and painlessly.[7]

* * *

The mind's influence on our physical health is well documented in the research from psychoneuroimmunology (PNI). P refers to psych, the mind; N the nervous system; and I the immune system. PNI research has clearly shown that the mind, nervous system, and immunological systems interact. Hope and positive belief can promote healing. Lack of hope and feelings of helplessness can lead to death. We can even talk to our T-cells, a form of biofeedback, to help us deal with bacteria in infections, viruses, and cancer. T-cells are important fighters in the body's response to foreign cells.(see Appendix A).[8]

Especially in health care, how the listener understands the content of what is said is more important than the content itself. The intended consequences of what is said may be very different from what one expects.

When the pediatrician listened to Mrs. Hurlburt's story he realized her thoughts and anxiety were understandable. Why, indeed, would the professor say that her son's hydrocephalus was arrested when he continued to see him every three months. It was predictable that the psychiatrist was unable to resolve this situation by only reassuring and prescribing medication for her. How, indeed, could she accept his reassurances when the issue was not being addressed, namely that the professor's reassurances didn't match his treatment schedule. The pediatrician understood that the mixed message that led to her anxious concern needed to be addressed. Since her son's hydrocephalus had not progressed, and he found nothing remarkable on his examination, he decided to check him less often. The treatment plan finally matched her son's condition. Problem resolved.

Verify, verify, emphasized Orlando. You haven't responded to the need until you verify what the need is, then verify that your response met that need. If the need is adequately responded to the behavior changes for the better.

The clinic patient in her forties was startled when she heard the eminent Dr. Samuel Levine say TS to his cardiology trainees as he finished examining her. She could not be persuaded by Dr. Lown that TS did not mean terminal situation, that it only meant tricuspid stenosis, not life threatening at all. After all, she had known Dr. Levine since her childhood when rheumatic fever had brought her to him. She revered and relied on him because he had saved her through many previous medical situations. Dr. Lown tried to resolve the situation by carefully explaining the meaning of the term. She could not accept anything other than what she believed her eminent doctor meant. At least Dr. Lown called Dr. Levine to come and resolve the situation. Unfortunately he did not believe it was as serious as Dr. Lown related. Dr. Levine assumed the situation could wait until he saw her that evening after his private patient rounds. Not so. Too late. She dies.

Even though Dr. Lown had been through the previous situation as a trainee, later when he was a cardiologist with his own staff, he didn't realize that the patient whose heart showed a wholesome gallop might misunderstand that term. The patient was at death's door with a heart almost completely destroyed in a severe heart attack with many complications. But this patient misunderstands in his favor. He believes his heart must be healthy. He lives.

Mr. Wright believes Krebiozen is his last hope. His health gets better or worse as he believes or not in the medicine. Yet again we see an example of how words from a doctor whom we respect and trust can be critical, especially when we are seriously ill. The woman who had improved from cancer with laetrile treatment in Mexico was doing fine until the doctor she had originally seen pronounced that treatment quackery. Poignant words for her. She died that night.

The last two stories are endearing as much because of the warm relationship between the patients and their doctors as for the outcomes. It is remarkable that Tony lives twelve years beyond the diagnosis of end stage cardiomyopathy by positively responding to his doctor's two five-year contracts. He believed and trusted in his doctor's expertise, therefore the contracts worked, but also because he clearly wanted and needed to live longer. Marrying and having a few years with his young mistress was clearly important to him. Dr. Kronberg gives Joe a reason to live when he prescribes "One set of memoirs." Joe survives until he finishes his manuscript and can present it to his beloved doctor. Then together they work out a plan for him to die as peacefully as possible.

Our histories, beliefs, expectations, and how we are experiencing our health or that of our families, affects how we hear our doctors. Because we are dependent on the doctors who examine and treat us, they need to realize that how we hear and understand what they say about our illnesses and treatments can be crucial to whether and how we revive, survive, or die.

14. When We Are Patients

The wind and heavily falling snow relentlessly hitting my face made me squint as I opened the door to Yale University Health. I stamped my feet on the mat, shook the snow off my jacket, and, with my right eye closed, half stumbled as I turned toward what appeared to be walk-in admissions. I gave the requested information and stated that every time I blinked or moved my right eye, there was a scratching sensation. I added that I had not been able to find anything in that eye.

Within a few minutes a young, dark haired physician was peering into my right eye with a small focused light. He pulled my eyelid back and told me to move my eye left and right, then up and down. To his questions I told him the scratching sensation was there every time I blinked or looked around. He asked me to do it again, and again, and kept asking me if I felt anything different. "No," I said. "The scratching sensation hasn't changed. Actually, it feels worse." "I don't see anything," he stated. "I couldn't either," I said, "but the scratching feeling is still there." He stood up. He looked off somewhere, then looked down at me. "Well, I can't find anything," he said with emphasis. "Well, it hasn't changed," I said with even more emphasis. He responded with silence and again looked off somewhere. He looked as if he were going to dismiss me.

"Please listen," I said. He turned and sternly looked down at me. "I'm not a hypochondriac. I'm a faculty member at the Medical Center." My words poured out as he stared at me with a slight frown. "I have a very busy schedule. I wouldn't be here unless something were wrong. I'm supposed to fly to Florida tomorrow to spend some time with my folks. I can't get on the plane and leave here with my eye like this." More silence from him. He looked up, then abruptly walked away, leaving me sitting there. I was dumbfounded.

A few minutes later he returned. With the same stern expression he stared down at me. "Take the elevator to the second floor. Someone there will see you." About as soon as he spoke, he turned and left. I got up, found the elevator, and took it to the second floor. As the elevator door opened, a matronly, middle aged woman who was standing there looked at me and, with a quizzical inflection, said my name. I responded with a nod. She immediately waved for me to follow her.

In a very small office she motioned me to sit in the ophthalmology chair. She picked up a magnifying scope and turned on its piercing light. "When did your eye start hurting?" She spoke clearly and kindly. She had leaned over toward me and was now looking into my eye with the lighted scope. "I think it started when I took my shower last night. I went to bed immediately afterward, but barely noticed it then. It's really been bothering me since I got up this morning."

She kept looking into my eye. I felt a quick prick. "Blink your eye. Does it hurt now?" she asked. "No," I said. "I don't feel the scratch any more." She nodded with satisfaction and turned off the lighted scope. "You had a very tiny, almost invisible, eyelash that had gone under your eyelid. I think it happened when you took your shower. I've pulled it out. It won't bother you any more." The tweezers were still in her hand.

"I can't thank you enough. I'm very grateful." Her gentle, sure manner, her focused question regarding when the symptom began, her skill in swiftly removing the errant eyelash, all of which so quickly solved the problem, made me want to hug her. As I left the office I looked at her, nodded, and smiled. She responded with a soft smile and nod, then quickly turned and walked down the hall.

As I took the elevator to the first floor and walked out into the snowstorm I realized I had never considered when my eye first began to bother me until the question was asked. My answer offered relevant information. Even with that information, since the eyelash was almost invisible, the first physician without the ophthalmology equipment may not have found it. However, I resolved to be more conscientious in including such information for physicians in the future. Oh yes, since then when taking a shower I do not let the water hit my face without closing my eyes.

* * *

When surgeon Pamela Gallin, M.D., needed surgery on her right hand, the hand she operates with, she chose one of the world's best hand surgeons, a respected academic physician who trained world famous surgeons. The procedure went well. The next day she returned home with her hand in a cast and an appointment to be seen in six weeks. She thought she had a high pain threshold, but, because she was having unbearable pain, she took a narcotic. Nothing changed, so she called her surgeon and told him she was in a lot of pain. He reassured her she was fine, and promised that the pain would go away. The pain worsened. So, for three more days she called, stated her situation, but still was not given an appointment. By then her fingers had swollen and looked like sausages.

Given the agony, she knew she was not fine. A radiologist friend told her to demand to be seen. This time she telephoned her surgeon's office and said she wanted to be seen. His secretary told her that her surgeon was out of town. She said she didn't care, she'd see someone else. So she saw another surgeon, another professor. She commented about his care. "He looked at my hand and literally ripped the cast off. Though he didn't say anything, I could tell he was furious. At that moment, I realized I wasn't being unreasonable."

She had not known how much pain to expect, but the severe pain and swelling had indeed indicated something was terribly wrong. A too tight cast had remained on for five days. The top of it had been pressing down across the base of her hand which resulted in impeding the blood supply and crushing the nerves. When the cast was taken off, not only was there swelling, the incision had popped open. Ultimately she saw a neurologist who confirmed that she had nerve damage in the skin of her hand. It took six months for the nerves to grow back. For the next two years she underwent two scar revisions by a plastic surgeon who specialized in hands. Each time she was in a cast for a month.

In retrospect she believed she should have not taken the narcotic for the initial pain, that it had masked the seriousness of the problem. She also thought that if she, a surgeon, were too intimidated to confront her doctor when she sensed something was wrong, then it must be more difficult for persons not familiar with or involved in health care to speak up when someone in authority is questioning them. She admitted that her surgeon's lack of response made her feel she was a bad patient. She encourages any of us to speak up to be seen when we feel something is wrong, and refuse to take no for an answer.

She also added the following. "But much of what I went through—days of excruciating pain, persisting nerve damage, the inconvenience and expense of subsequent surgery—would not have happened had the surgeon listened to me and treated me with respect."[1]

* * *

Ellen O'Connor is a soft spoken data processor in her late twenties who is known for her ready smile. Michael, her husband, is a salesman. A pediatrician sent Ellen with Sandra, their six-month-old daughter, to the hospital emergency room because he was concerned that Sandra's fever and diarrhea might indicate that she had intussusception (one part of the intestine telescopes into another, causing obstruction). An intern examined her. He obtained X-rays of her abdomen which he believed suggested an internal blockage leading him to say that she needed exploratory surgery. Ellen asked him if he thought, or knew this. The intern did not respond with a straight answer.

Ellen and Michael waited several hours for the results of their daughter's blood tests and for the surgical team to assemble. During those hours Sandra felt less feverish to her mother, and she was no longer cranky. She had become calm. So Ellen told the intern that Sandra had become more like her usual self. Ellen shook her head as she later talked about how the intern didn't listen. He kept insisting that Sandra be taken for surgery. Ellen and Michael held fast. They refused to have Sandra taken to surgery when her symptoms had improved. After much argument, the intern told the parents they would have to sign a legal release assuming responsibility for their decision if they refused to have Sandra taken to the operating room. Ellen later commented. "I'm not a doctor or a nurse. But I'm a mother, and I know my child, and I felt deep inside that she was okay."

Ellen asked the intern what other tests could prove his suspicion of intussusception. He said an ultrasound, but it was expensive and would require a specialist to come in to do the test. Ellen stayed firm and made it clear that in no way would she back down about the surgery. She said the ultrasound specialist who was called to come in gave them a really hard time. To the surprise of the doctors the ultrasound showed no intussusception. Sandra's intestines were moving normally. She had viral gastroenteritis, an infection. Ellen admitted: "It was a hard decision for people like us to question the doctors. But we needed to be sure they were right. It was my baby."[2]

* * *

Jerome Groopman, M.D., developed a nagging ache in his right hip when training for the Boston Marathon. He believed he had bursitis. A sports medicine doctor prescribed anti-inflammatory medication for the presumed bursitis and supported his request to exercise on a rowing machine, but only for light rowing. Instead, Dr. Groopman rowed with the oars at high resistance and ignored the progressively worsening dull ache in his hip. Within a few minutes a viselike spasm exploded in his lower back accompanied by the feeling that electric shocks were speeding down his legs. He fell to the floor and for many hours remained there in a fetal position until the pain eased. Finally he hobbled to bed. His wife, also a physician, then a resident at the Massachusetts General Hospital in Boston, suggested strict bed rest, continued anti-inflammatory medication, and time.

However, Dr. Groopman wanted an immediate solution. He went to various doctors until he found a neurosurgeon who told him what he wanted to hear. He accepted a limited operation on what had now been diagnosed as a bulging disc. Results of the surgery were no better. He was left with a dull ache in his back and hip. Less than a year from the first nagging ache he stood up, then abruptly collapsed. As before, a powerful spasm gripped his lower back. Again it felt as if electric shocks were racing down his legs. X-rays showed no clear reason for this relapse. No bulging discs were detected. So he consulted rheumatologists, neurosurgeons, and sports medicine doctors. All of them said that the lumbar spine is a black box and is best left alone to heal itself. But Dr. Groopman was still unwilling to believe that passive healing was the answer. He wanted a clear diagnosis and an immediate and permanent solution.

He found an orthopedist who told him he had instability of his lower spine and suggested a fusion. Bone would be harvested from his pelvis and inserted along the ridges of his lower spine. That would create an internal brace and fully restore his mobility. The orthopedist's partner, a neurosurgeon, was not so optimistic.

However, Dr. Groopman went ahead with the surgery. When he awoke in the intensive care unit he found that moving his legs or just flexing his toes would trigger waves of enormous pain. He learned that he had hemorrhaged during the operation. He had been cleared for the surgery, but it was possible that the previous anti-inflammatory medication had weakened his blood's ability to clot. The agony didn't subside. He was told he had neuritis, that his spinal nerves had been irritated from the spilled blood and from scarring.

The orthopedist offered another operation to free the nerves. Dr. Groopman's wife insisted he decline. This time he accepted her advice. For three months he lay on ice to numb the stabbing pain. The strong medication prescribed for the pain left him nauseated and unable to focus, think, or read. He became despondent. He finally consulted a specialist in rehabilitation medicine. Even with physical therapy it took almost a year for him to walk more than a few yards.

He has never fully recovered. Because of the limits on his functioning, no day passes without his thinking of his headstrong decision to agree to the surgery. In retrospect he believes that the original ache in his hip wasn't bursitis, but referred pain from a nerve pinched by a bulging lumbar disc. He finally realized that his desperate belief in a perfect solution was a fantasy.[5]

* * *

Atul Gawande, M.D., remembers the following situation from his hospital internship year. Mr. Howe, in his late thirties, was in the hospital recovering from surgery for a severely infected gallbladder. Three days after the surgery he spiked a high fever. His heart raced over a hundred beats a minute. His blood pressure was too low and he was short of breath. Even with the maximum oxygen flow in his oxygen mask, his blood showed barely adequate oxygen levels.

His face was flushed, he was sweating profusely, his eyes were wide opened, and he was panting as he sat bent forward propped up on his arms. His operative incision showed no signs of infection. He denied pain in his abdomen. But when Dr. Gawande listened to Mr. Howe's lungs through a stethoscope, his lungs sounded like a washing machine. Even with the oxygen flowing at maximum level, Mr. Howe kept struggling to breathe. Mr. Howe's wife, a small, thin, pale woman, stood nearby, rocking on her feet, hugging herself.

Mr. Howe was on intravenous fluids which included antibiotics. Dr. Gawande drew blood for tests and cultures, then paged a chief resident whom he knew. She immediately returned his call. He filled her in on the details and told her he needed her help. Without delay the chief resident came into the room. She was just past thirty years old, almost six feet tall, athletic in appearance, and had a no-nonsense manner. She looked at Mr. Howe and murmured to the nurse to keep an intubation kit available near his bed. She put her hand on Mr. Howe's shoulder and asked him how he was. "Fine," he finally answered after he had caught a breath. She explained that it was likely that he had pneumonia, and it probably would be getting worse. She told him antibiotics would not immediately solve the problem, and it was obvious he was tiring out quickly. To get him through this, she said, she needed to put him to sleep, intubate him, and put him on a breathing machine.

"No," he sat straight up and gasped, "Don't . . . put me . . . on a . . . machine." She told him it might only be for a couple of days. He'd be given sedatives so he'd be as comfortable as possible. She wanted to be sure he understood that he'd die without the ventilator. Shaking his head he emphasized, "No . . . machine!" Dr. Gawande and the chief resident knew Mr. Howe had reason to live. He had a wife and a child. He was young and otherwise healthy. They wondered if fear or lack of understanding was influencing his decision. They believed antibiotics and high-tech support would pull him through.

The chief resident looked at Mrs. Howe and asked her what she thought her husband should do. She looked stricken with fear. "I don't know, I don't know," she answered as she burst into tears. "Can't you save him?" Unable to tolerate the situation anymore, Mrs. Howe left the room. When the chief resident realized her attempts to persuade Mr. Howe were of no use, she left and phoned his attending surgeon at home. Then she returned and waited until Mr. Howe tired out. Pale and sweaty, oxygen levels dropping, he closed his eyes and gradually became unconscious.

The chief resident immediately went into action. She lowered Mr. Howe's bed until he lay flat. She instructed a nurse to put a tranquilizing medication into his intravenous fluids. She put a mask over his face and squeezed breaths of oxygen into his lungs. Dr. Gawande handed her the intubation equipment. On the first try she slipped a long, clear plastic breathing tube down into his trachea. The two physicians wheeled him in his bed to the elevator, then down a few floors to the intensive care unit. Later Dr. Gawande found Mrs. Howe and explained that her husband was on a ventilator in the intensive care unit. Saying nothing, she went to intensive care to see him.

Over the next twenty-four hours Mr. Howe's lungs markedly improved. Sedation was reduced and he was able to take over breathing from the machine. He didn't struggle when he opened his eyes with the breathing tube sticking out of his mouth. He nodded when Dr. Gawande asked permission to remove the tube. Dr. Gawande cut the ties, deflated the balloon cuff that held the tube in place, and pulled it out. Mr. Howe coughed briefly, but violently.

Dr. Gawande quietly stood there looking at Mr. Howe. "You had pneumonia, but you're doing just fine now." He felt anxious waiting for his patient's response. Mr. Howe winced from the soreness in his throat and swallowed hard. Then he looked at Dr. Gawande, and in a hoarse yet steady voice said, "Thank you."[4]

* * *

It was mid-November when seventy-nine-year-old Jeffrey Butler, a retired Wesleyan University professor from Middletown, Connecticut, collapsed on the kitchen floor from a stroke. He was never one to give up. Though he had lost his left arm in World War II, he had built bookcases for the living room. He had a Ph.D. from Oxford, had coached rugby, and with his two sons had sailed on Long Island Sound. Jeffrey and his wife, Valerie, had been active. They walked daily. He was writing a history of his birthplace, a small South African town. Now their lives were irreparably disrupted.

Six weeks after his stroke Jeffrey returned home, permanently incapable of completing a sentence. He doggedly moved forward. He learned how to fasten his belt, peck out sentences on his computer, and, with one foot dragging, walk by himself to the university pool for water aerobics. But he needed help to put on his shirt, and he no longer continued writing his book. Despite his difficulty speaking, in a halting voice he told his wife, "I don't know who I am anymore."

His stroke devastated their lives. Valerie became a frustrated and exhausted caretaker. When she saw their internist, Dr. Fales, she burst into tears. He put her on antidepressants and sleeping pills. The following fall, one year after his stroke, in his garbled speech he told Katy, his daughter, that her mother would have been better off if he had died.

Just before Christmas, after vigorous water exercises, Jeffrey Butler developed a painful inguinal hernia. Dr. Fales sent him to a local surgeon who sent him to a cardiologist to evaluate and clear him for surgery. Because Jeffrey had a slow heartbeat, Dr. Rogan, the cardiologist, would not clear him for surgery without a pacemaker. Dr. Rogan later told Katy that her father could otherwise have died from cardiac arrest during surgery. About a year before, Jeffrey had seen Dr. Rogan who had suggested a pacemaker for the same slow heartbeat. Then, on the advice of Dr. Fales, Jeffrey had refused. Slow heartbeats can be unremarkable, longstanding, and common in old folks.

This time Jeffrey Butler was too mentally incapacitated from his stroke to discuss whether or not to have the pacemaker, so, as his health care proxy, the decision fell to his wife. She was deferential to doctors, exhausted, and anxious to relieve her husband's pain. Despite his having refused a pacemaker earlier, she consented.

Dr. Fales received the news by fax. If he had been given the opportunity to discuss this with the Butlers, he could have told them that a pacemaker's battery can last ten years. He could have asked if Jeffrey wanted to live to age eighty-nine in his debilitated state. He could have told them there was an option of having a temporary external pacemaker that could have supported him through the surgery.

Soon after the new year Valerie telephoned Katy with the news that her father had come through the pacemaker insertion and hernia repair without any problem. However, the struggles at home continued. Some two years more the age-related degeneration that had slowed his heart now affected his eyes, lungs, bladder, and bowels. He became incontinent. He began losing his sight to macular degeneration which resulted in ocular injections costing nearly $2,000 each. Within three more years he fell in the driveway from a brain hemorrhage. "The Jeff I married . . . is no longer the same person," Valerie wrote in a journal a social worker had suggested she keep.

On the internet Katy learned that pacemakers could be deactivated without surgery. If nothing were done, her father's pacemaker might not stop for years. Four and a half years after the pacemaker and hernia surgery Valerie asked Dr. Rogan to deactivate the pacemaker. He was morally opposed, and refused. Soon thereafter she declined additional medical tests and refused to have her husband put on a new drug for dementia and a blood thinner with problematic side effects. In her journal she wrote, "Enough of all this overkill! It's killing me! Talk about quality of life—what about mine?"

Jeffrey Butler began to yell at his caregivers, and he and Valerie began shouting at each other. He was not sick enough to be admitted to hospice care, but he was sick enough to never get better. Finally he was weak enough to qualify for palliative care which allowed for nurses and social workers to visit at home. Shortly thereafter he was hospitalized for pneumonia. Valerie begged her husband's doctors and nurses to increase his morphine dose and to turn off the pacemaker. The doctor on call at Dr. Rogan's cardiology practice refused authorization to deactivate the pacemaker because he "might die immediately." Katy began to draft an appeal to the hospital ethics committee. For five days she and her mother took shifts to sit by his bedside as his breathing became ragged and they watched his body slowly fail. Now, in his mid-eighties, with his pacemaker continuing to beat in his chest, Jeffrey Butler finally stopped breathing.

A year later, Valerie Butler, now eighty-four, was diagnosed with two leaking heart valves. She was offered open heart surgery. She was told that without the surgery there was a fifty-fifty chance she would die within two years. If she survived the operation she probably would live to age ninety. The surgeon would not accept do-not-resuscitate if they needed to revive her during surgery. He said it would not be fair to his team. In tears she told him, "If I have a stroke I want you to let me go." He countered by telling her there was the possibility that she might have only a minor stroke, just some weakness on one side. Then he sent her to another floor for an echocardiogram. A half-hour later she returned. She made clear she would not submit to the surgery. Emphatically she announced, "I will not do it."

That spring and summer Valerie Butler arranged for house repairs, pitched the files that her husband had been working with to write his book, and cleaned out his bookcases. She didn't want to leave a mess for her children. In August she had a heart attack and returned home with hospice care. A month later she had another heart attack. She was admitted to the hospice wing of the hospital. The next morning she took off her silver earrings. She had remained continent. She was lucid. She told the nurses she wanted to stop eating and drinking. She said she wanted to die and never go home. An hour later Valerie Butler died.[5]

* * *

When we are patients, whether we realize it or not, we enter a relationship with our doctors that is influenced by our expectations and beliefs. We may be wary if we have had miserable experiences. We may expect a reasonable, understanding, and skillful response if our previous encounters have been helpful. We may be surprised if what we experience is different from what we expect. Because we are dependent on our doctors to reasonably respond to us with our ills, and because we don't fully know what will happen in that process, we also enter those relationships with some anxiety.

What we, and they, may fail to fully realize, is the crucial importance of the relationship itself. It is through that relationship that each understands the other. For a successful outcome, each needs to understand the other. As we have seen in these stories, misunderstandings and differences of opinions can lead to problematic outcomes. Our doctors, like us, enter each relationship and each encounter with their own expectations and beliefs. Their expectations and beliefs may be the same as ours, or they may be different. These differences may or may not be easily understood or, if understood, accepted. Resolving the situations may include intense confrontations, and the result may or may not be satisfactory to either or both sides.

There are situations where some doctors dismiss what we say. They may even dismiss us. It certainly appeared to me that the doctor who was unable to discover the cause for my scratchy eye was considering dismissing me. I had to emphasize that I had a problem that needed to be solved. As a surgeon, Pam Gallin, M.D., believed that the post operative excruciating pain in her hand needed to be addressed, yet for three days her surgeon dismissed her over the phone. He would not see her. Given the increased agony, combined with the continually increasing swelling in her fingers, she finally demanded to be seen. Since she, as a surgeon, had been too intimidated to confront her doctor, she wondered how much more difficult it must be for the average patient.

Ellen O'Connor and her husband were confronted with an intern with an obstinate, dogged belief that could not easily be shaken. Though he would not state whether he just thought or really believed that the X-rays of their daughter's abdomen really showed intussusception, he moved forward in his plan to assemble a surgical team to do exploratory surgery. He was not swayed by the evidence that their daughter's symptoms were improving, and made it clear they'd have to sign a release if they didn't allow her to have the operation. Only when Ellen asked him if there were any tests that might give them the needed information did he admit that ultrasound was such a test. Even then he balked at calling in the ultrasound specialist. Ellen had to stay firm in wanting the non-invasive ultrasound over the invasive exploratory surgery.

Jerome Groopman, M.D., as patient, was looking for a permanent fix for a complicated, painful, neurological back problem. He would not be dismissed. He went to various doctors until they said what he wanted to hear. Even after unsuccessful surgery he found another surgeon willing to operate. He went ahead despite many consultants having told him that the lumbar spine is best left alone to heal itself. After the second surgery left him in an even worse state, he finally accepted his physician wife's insistence that he seek no further surgery. He has never fully recovered. He admitted he was too headstrong, that his desperate belief in a perfect solution had been a fantasy.

In Mr. Howe's situation the chief resident dismissed his utterance of no machine. She believed his healthy history and current acute illness warranted extreme measures to save him. She and Dr. Gawande were not sure he was capable of fully understanding his situation. So she turned to his terrified wife who made it clear she wanted her husband saved. Extreme measures were taken. Mr. Howe was saved and responded with "thank you."

The situation with Jeffrey and Valerie Butler is one any of us may eventually face. After his stroke, Jeffrey refused a pacemaker. Later, when he was incapable of answering rationally, Valerie, as his health care proxy, had to answer the same question. The specialist would not operate and repair Jeffrey's hernia without one. Deferential to doctors, exhausted, and anxious to relieve her husband's pain, she accepted a permanent pacemaker. She was not told a temporary pacemaker could be used during the operation. Her internist knew this, but was not included in the discussion. The repair was successful. His post stroke, downhill course with increasing dementia continued. Valerie begged to have the pacemaker deactivated. The on call cardiologist refused, saying her husband might die. Finally she and her daughter took shifts by his bedside watching his body fail. He died with the pacemaker continuing to beat in his chest. After all this Valerie decided to handle her final years differently. Her surgeon refused to accept do-not-resuscitate if his team needed to revive her during recommended surgery for leaking heart valves, so she refused the surgery. She put her life in order and, fully aware, with the support of hospice and her family, she died peacefully.

These stories of patients who are mentally aware, or who have health care proxies who can speak for them, minimally highlight the following: we need to state our symptoms as succinctly as possible, include when they occurred and, if possible, why we think they occurred. Expect to be physically examined. Lisa Sanders, M.D., comments that the patient's story, combined with a physical examination, can lead the physician to possible diagnoses or to specific tests that might be needed. She is aware that some physicians will go directly to tests which, if the physical examination were done, may not be needed.[6] If an invasive procedure is suggested, such as exploratory surgery, ask if there is a non-invasive way to get the same information.

Neither we nor our information should be dismissed. If necessary, demand to be heard and evaluated. Know ahead of time where to go in an emergency. We deserve to be treated with respect and understanding. We have the final decision as to what we will accept. Our health care proxies should understand what we will accept if their input is needed. As such, advance directives should be in place and available, even though they do not cover all possible situations. Do know that doctors may say they won't agree to accept them under some circumstances. We saw that in the Jeffrey Butler story.

From his writing and teaching at the Yale University Law School, Jay Katz, M.D., believes that "physicians and patients must share the burdens of decision," and that "the choices of all but incompetent individuals must be honored." He also notes that "studies have shown that patients evaluate care more favorably and have better outcomes when they feel their physicians have genuinely communicated with them."[7]

From his research, Attorney Carl E. Schneider, University of Michigan Law School, notes that patients have two main criteria about their doctors. They want competent and caring doctors. He also believes that "patients have no unvarying duty to make medical decisions. Rather, the question what role to take will often be problematic for all concerned, will vary vastly from case to case and time to time."[8]

Most important, build a relationship with a primary care physician who is competent, who listens, and who cares. When we are patients we should never assume what will occur. We should be sure we are telling our stories as succinctly as possible. We need to be sure our physicians are on our wavelengths, and we on theirs. We need to understand each other in order to make rational decisions. After all, it is our lives we are talking about, not theirs.

15. Hospitals

It was 8:00 a.m. and I had just arrived at my local hospital for day surgery. My husband had given me a ride and was walking into the Day Care Surgery Unit with me. I was scheduled for a cataract operation, but I was not looking forward to it. Generally speaking, we health care professionals don't much like being patients. We know too much and don't welcome being put in a dependent position.

I was the first patient to arrive. A few staff looked up, as did the charge nurse whom I recognized. As colleagues we had been in a few situations together. She nodded with a smile, then introduced me to the nurse who would be with me. I introduced them to my husband who left after he understood that he could return to get me in about two hours. He wished me good luck, then turned and disappeared down the hallway toward the door.

Immediately various events began to occur. From my nurse: "Here's your gown, I'll put your clothes in this cabinet." Then she oriented me to the immediate treatment plan. In step by step fashion, as she started an intravenous infusion then administered eye drops, she explained what she would be doing and why. We chatted amiably. She encouraged me to ask questions, use the bathroom if needed, and express any concerns or needs. When she was involved elsewhere she often glanced over to see how I was. Periodically she came over to check on me and administer more eye drops. The chief nurse, nursing staff, and the physicians who wandered through conferred, as needed, in a professional, easy manner.

My ophthalmologist came in and asked me how I was doing. "Fine," I answered with a nod. Then the anesthesiologist came over and introduced himself. He asked a number of medical questions which I easily answered, and otherwise checked my chart's information regarding my status for the forthcoming operation. He acknowledged my understanding that I was to have a sedative. I told him this was important to me because I wanted as little sedation as possible so as to lessen the possibility of side effects. He concurred. He was cordial with an easy, sure manner. He checked the intravenous to be sure it was dripping as he wished and that the fluid was properly going into my vein. All this instilled confidence. Therefore I had no hesitation in giving in to the sedation. I was only barely aware of being rolled down to the operating room.

The next thing I remembered was being vaguely aware of some red and white colors, and I heard my ophthalmologist say, "It's perfect." I awoke back in the Day Care Surgery Unit where my nurse soon offered me a choice of drinks. When I started to drink the orange juice quickly, she put up her hand. "Not so fast." I gave her a questioning look. "Take it slow," she said. "You want to be sure to keep it down." I nodded and slowed down. She offered something to eat. I declined. "We want you to eat something." Since she was watching out for my welfare, I accepted one of her choices. She soon brought a warm, delicious piece of buttered toast. By now this large room was bustling with other patients and their staff, all under the watchful eye of the chief nurse who was overseeing this busy unit with confidence, efficiency, and relevant humor.

I requested to use the bathroom, and added "Can you remove the intravenous?" "No, I'll take it with you," my nurse responded as she helped me out of bed, walked with me, then hitched up the bag of fluid in the bathroom. After a reasonable interval she returned, knocked on the door, and walked me back to my bed. She understood that I was doing well, so she took out the intravenous.

After I changed back into my clothes and acknowledged my husband who had returned, the charge nurse signed me out with specific post operative instructions and a warm goodbye. "No, you're not allowed to walk. Hospital rules," said my nurse when she came over with a wheelchair which I tried to decline. She took me to the exit in the wheelchair while my husband retrieved his truck to drive me home. I thanked her and told her how impressed I was with her and the staff, and said that the experience was easier than I had expected. We waved each other a friendly good bye.

Now, only two hours later and comfortably in my husband's warm truck, I plugged in my seat belt, looked at him, and grinned. "Piece of cake. Couldn't have been easier." "Good," he said with a nod. "Let's go home."

* * *

Larry Kirkland, a physician and a paraplegic, was transferred to an intermediate care hospital for wound care after surgery for a deep pressure ulcer. His stay lasted sixteen days.

To treat the anemia which had developed from an infection secondary to the ulcer, he was put on ferrous sulfate three times a day. Since he knew it can irritate one's stomach, he requested the nurse to put the pill on the table for him to take during his meal which had just arrived. "I can't do that," she said. She picked up the cup with the pill. "I'll wait until you are ready." This was not a prescription drug. So he told her to cancel the order. He had his wife bring some ferrous sulfate tablets from home.

He had a Swiss Army type pocketknife with a two-and-a-quarter-inch blade, screwdriver, bottle opener, can opener, and awl. Given his limitations, he relied on this multi-purpose tool and always kept it within easy reach. When a nurse spied it on the bedside table she immediately said, "You can't have that in here." So he said he'd keep it out of sight. He thought that had solved the problem. However, later that day a woman in a business suit he believed was from administration, with a woman who seemed to be there as a witness, went straight to the bedside table, opened the drawer, and removed the pocketknife. As she left she said it would be locked in a safe place. She gave him no chance to reply.

A night nurse woke him at 6:00 a.m. to take his temperature. Since he had no fever, this could have waited a few hours. He asked her to write on the chart "patient refused." She said this had to be done before her shift ended at 7:00 a.m. She told him she knew someone who was laid off for not doing something similar. She added that when she was hired she was told she had to go along with the way things were done. If she could not, she should look for another job. So he conceded and let her take his temperature. Also, he had to accept nurses cursorily listening to his chest on every shift even though he was alert, had no fever, no chest symptoms, and no coughs. As a physician he knew that this offered no valuable information. Only once did a temporary weekend registered nurse have him sit up and roll over to listen to his lungs, the proper procedure.

When some of the staff realized that he continually questioned policies and regulations he deemed nonsensical, he was labeled a problem patient. He realized this when a woman who said she was from "bed assignment" told him she had phoned about the possibility of his being transferred back to the hospital where he'd had his surgery. This, however, did not happen.

The above were only some of the rules and regulations he was expected to accept. Even the page system which was above the head of his bed blared questions or messages not directly related to patients' individual needs. A typical question was: "Jane, do you have the keys?"

He made the following statement about his care. "As a physician and as a patient, I'd never before come across so many staff members seemingly fearful of using their own experience, common sense and judgment in making a decision, nor so many who cited 'policy' or 'regulations' to explain a particular action."[1]

Maybe, like the nurse who was told to comply or go elsewhere, they feared losing their jobs.

* * *

During her training, Dr. Karen Delgado was on duty in a busy hospital emergency room in the wee hours of the morning. The police had brought in a young man whom they had found sleeping on the steps of a local art museum. She noted that he was unshaven, had on dirty clothes, was uncooperative, and apparently unwilling to rouse himself. He did not respond clearly to questions from the triage nurse. Dr. Delgado was very busy attending other patients, so she eyeballed him and decided to leave him on a gurney in the corridor. Since it was the 1970s, she thought he was another homeless hippie. They would give him breakfast in the morning and return him to the streets.

Some hours later a nurse was tugging at her sleeve. "I really want you to go back and examine that guy," said the nurse with some urgency. Dr. Delgado was reluctant because she felt she was involved with more demanding concerns. However, she had learned to respect emergency room nurses who believed that something was seriously wrong with any of their patients.

A blood test showed that this man's blood sugar was sky-high. He was heading into a diabetic coma. Because he had been too weak and lethargic to get back to his apartment, he had fallen asleep on the art museum steps. He was a student, not a vagrant.

His struggle to give the police and the triage nurse information were due to the metabolic changes that typify out-of-control diabetes.

After that experience, Dr. Delgado said she would conjure up the picture of that young man whenever she was called to the emergency room to evaluate a disheveled and uncooperative patient. "The hardest thing about being a doctor is that you learn best from your mistakes, mistakes made on living people," she said. She added: "It is impossible to catalogue all of the stereotypes that you carry in your mind." She believes that patients and their families need to be aware that doctors rely on pattern recognition and stereotypes to make decisions. She encourages patients and their families to diplomatically call their doctors' attention to incorrect interpretations when it is obvious to them that this is occurring.[2]

* * *

As a busy author, Norman Cousins was often working on various projects. In the last three months of 1980 he traveled almost constantly. He returned from a trip and discovered that he was supposed to take another trip in a few days. He asked his secretary about a postponement or cancellation. She reviewed the reasons that made it essential that he not cancel any of the engagements. The next day he had a heart attack. He was sixty-five years old.

A cardiogram revealed the scar of an old, previously unknown silent myocardial infarction, and the beginning of a new, more serious one. This time he also had congestive heart failure. He became a patient in a coronary care unit at the University of California Los Angeles Hospital.

He told his physician, Dr. Shine, that blood specimens were being drawn from him more than once a day. He requested Dr. Shine to have the involved departments coordinate and share in only one drawn blood a day. Dr. Shine agreed and authorized Norman to turn away any staff who were not following this agreement. Only once did Norman have to turn someone away. He also asked that hospital routines not take precedence over his need for sleep. At least could he please not be awakened during the night to be given medication. Dr. Shine also accepted this request and said he would so instruct the house staff.

The fourth night he couldn't sleep because he had a stuffy nose from a cold. So he asked the nurse for a nebulizer. When she asked if he had difficulty breathing he answered "yes." Instead of giving him time to explain, she abruptly left. Almost immediately a crew led by the resident in charge roared into his room. They flicked on the lights and began to put him on a rolling stretcher. He was told he was going to X-ray, and that he needed a cardiogram. It was 2:30 a.m. Norman told the resident that his problem with breathing was in his nose, not his chest. He just wanted something to open his sinuses so he could breathe more easily and get some sleep. Norman also knew they were interfering with the rest that he had been told was essential. They would not listen. Norman was furious. He sat up and ordered the entire crew out of the room. The resident backed off but said, "I'm going to call Dr. Shine." Norman shot back, "For heaven's sake, don't wake up the poor man." "But we've got to follow the rules!" emphasized the resident. "Doctor," said Norman, "I don't presume to tell you what to do, but one of the first things a doctor has to learn is when the rules don't apply. Now, you had better leave before you create the very situation you think you have to treat."

They did call Dr. Shine. He told them they could safely assume that Norman Cousins knew the difference between a stuffy nose and congestive heart failure. About a half hour later an attendant brought a nebulizer which enabled him to breathe more easily.

Another night Norman felt some slight chest pressure. Dr. Shine had told him to take a nitroglycerin tablet when he felt any unusual chest symptoms. Norman rang for the nurse. She told him she could not give him the nitroglycerin because Dr. Shine had said he was not to have medication at night. Norman explained that this order was there because Dr. Shine had honored his request not to be awakened at night. She nodded but didn't budge. Orders were orders. Because of the persistence of the heaviness in his chest, he pressed the point. It was no use. Sheer exasperation led him to demand to see the resident in charge. The resident came and immediately provided the nitroglycerin. He listened to Norman's chest, took his blood pressure, and stayed long enough to be sure the nitroglycerin had worked.

After four days in the coronary care unit he was moved to a private room where he made rapid progress. He was able to return home after a total hospital stay of about three weeks.[3]

* * *

Doug, Diane Payne's husband, was severely ill in a hospital intensive care unit. Eight physicians were involved in his care. By the second day she could no longer communicate with him. He was sedated, and a respirator was breathing for him. The cardiologist told her Doug was doing reasonably well. But when the lung specialist breezed into the room and listened to Doug's chest with a stethoscope, he said, "He's not getting better. He's worse. He may die. Any questions?" She was too stunned to coherently respond.

Later the nephrologist told Diane that Doug's kidneys were failing and he needed dialysis. She told this doctor what the other two specialists had said. She hoped he could help her understand their comments. Instead he pressed her with questions about what their findings were, questions she could not answer. She felt overwhelmed. After he was gone she left the room because she knew she needed to communicate with his parents who were in Florida, and with his brother in New Jersey. When she returned a nurse in the intensive care unit somewhat indignantly told her she had been trying to find her because there were more doctors to see.

When the infectious disease specialist appeared, she begged him for information. Was Doug dying or holding his own. This doctor took time to explain that doctors only evaluate the organ system of their specialty. He explained that even though Doug's heart was doing reasonably well, his lungs and kidneys were failing. He was definitely in danger of dying. The specialists were not able to pull him through. After thirty-eight days in intensive care, Doug died.

With so many specialists involved in a situation such as this, especially when they are unwilling to answer questions that do not pertain to their specialty, Diane believes there should be a designated person who is able to talk with family members about the patient's overall condition.[4]

* * *

My experience with cataract surgery was quintessential Orlando. My nurse and I were in this together. She was on my wavelength, and I on hers. She oriented me as to what would occur and why. Whether or not she could meet any of my requests, she kept me informed, as needed. She was continually watching out for my welfare. Since I had to give up control during the operation, I wanted to know if my understanding that I would have a sedative was true. When the anesthesiologist validated that this was so, that information and his manner allowed me to give control over to him. I already had confidence in my ophthalmologist, or I would not have been there.

Orlando would call this excellent patient care. Never assume, she used to emphasize. This staff never assumed. I was given information as needed, communication was always kept clear, and requests allowed when reasonable. If you believe all this was possible because the charge nurse and I knew each other, not so. Other than my ophthalmologist, my second cataract operation a couple years later was with an entirely different staff, and my experience was essentially the same.

Rules and regulations ruled Larry Kirkland's patient experience. As a physician and patient, he had never seen so many staff who turned to policy or regulations to explain their actions, nor so many who seemed afraid to use their own experience, common sense, and judgment to make decisions. He was given no say and no control over what would happen. He was at the mercy of what the staff had been told to do. His patient experience was the antithesis of patient care that responds to individual patient needs.

Dr. Karen Delgado was pressed with the demands of a busy hospital emergency room. When the emergency room nurse realized that the patient they had left on the gurney needed an urgent reevaluation, Dr. Delgado immediately responded to the nurse's concerns. Later Dr. Delgado admitted with regret that she had initially, and too quickly, made the incorrect assumption that the unkempt young man was a vagrant. She was willing to recognize the mistake and learn from it. What is important is that she and the nurse communicated well with each other. They respected each other's ability to reevaluate the situation. As such they were able to resolve a crisis that was becoming worse. As patients we want and need our doctors and nurses to work well with each other, to be receptive to new information about a situation, to recognize when they are making assumptions, and to validate those assumptions for their accuracy.

Norman Cousins and his physician, Dr. Shine, had a relationship we would all hope to have with our doctors. Both respected each other's ability to ascertain what was needed and reasonable at any point in time. They were able to negotiate what was in Norman's best interest in order to keep as smooth as possible the healing process. Important to this process was Norman's ability to speak up and be heard, and Dr. Shine's ability to listen and be responsive to what reasonably could be allowed.

The night nurse too quickly assumed that Norman's difficulty with breathing was due to cardiac problems. She functioned automatically according to where they were, a coronary care unit, and according to her training and beliefs. Instead of giving Norman time to state why he thought he was having difficulty breathing, she swiftly left and alerted the resident who rushed in with his crew and began to take Norman for tests to evaluate his cardiac condition. Again Norman tried to explain that he only needed a nebulizer to relieve his stuffy nose so he could sleep. The resident and his crew still would not listen.

Only when Norman became furious, sat up, and ordered them out of the room did they retreat. They called Dr. Shine despite Norman's protests to not telephone and awaken "the poor man." The resident emphasized his rationale: "we've got to follow the rules!" In the phone conversation Dr. Shine supported Norman, and the nebulizer soon arrived.

The next situation with the nurse is similar. Because Dr. Shine's orders stated that Norman was not to receive medication at night, she refused to honor his request for nitroglycerine when he felt chest pressure. Ironically, nitroglycerin was exactly what Dr. Shine had told him to take under such circumstances. Out of sheer exasperation Norman again had to emphasize his need to be heard. He demanded to see the resident. This time he and the resident were able to resolve the situation without Dr. Shine being called. The resident provided the nitroglycerin and stayed to be sure it worked.

Diane's husband, Doug, was in a hospital intensive care unit so severely ill that he was involved with eight physicians. Like Norman, she had to beg to be heard. She needed to know whether her husband was dying or holding his own. Finally the infectious disease specialist listened and told her that her husband was in danger of dying, not a clear answer, but more than she had heard from any of the others.

When we are patients in hospitals or other inpatient health care facilities, we lose some independence. How much we lose depends on why we are there, our condition, our relationship with those responsible for our care and treatment, and to what degree the staff adhere to their institutional rules and regulations. Orlando believed that hospital patients' distress was sometimes more because of adverse reactions to the setting rather than to their reason for being there. This is certainly evident in some of these stories.

Good patient care involves having competent staff who are able to use reasonable judgment in patient situations. Good patient care means that the staff listen to and communicate well with their patients, and treat them as valuable members of the care team. When patients are conscious and able to be involved with their care, they can give valuable verbal data to assist in that care. Nonverbal data should of course be evaluated as needed.

When we are patients, it is not only doctors who need our stories to assist them in making accurate diagnoses and treatment plans. The other staff also need our stories and our nonverbal data to help them accurately respond to our needs. When we as patients realize they are not listening to us or are making incorrect assumptions about us, we need to speak up and be counted. It may be difficult but, as noted in the story about Norman Cousins, it may be essential.

16. Hospitals and Hierarchies

To Err is Human, an Institute of Medicine (IOM) Report published in 2000, estimated that between 44,000 and 98,000 patients died from medical errors in U.S. hospitals in 1997, exceeding the number of deaths from motor vehicle accidents, breast cancer, or AIDS. Though the IOM Report noted that the health care system itself can cause errors, it also noted that human error is one of the greatest contributors to accidents in any industry, including health care. This Report made many recommendations and stated that the ultimate goal of all their recommendations is to create safety systems by implementing safe practices at the delivery level. The Report recommended developing a working culture where communication flows freely throughout the system.[1]

Hospitals are hierarchical systems with people in rank order serving various functions within each system. Whether the hospital is a large metropolitan hospital or a small rural hospital, it usually has a Board of Trustees with some policy making responsibilities and a president with the authority to make major administrative decisions. Various administrative and clinical departments have their rank order staff who carry out their own various functions.

Though roles and responsibilities need to be clear, and policies and procedures need to be designed for patient safety, communication from the president on down, as well as within and between departments, may ultimately be one of the most critical components in delivering quality patient care. This includes the climate within which the communication occurs.

Though these stories highlight some of the communication issues within hospital systems, they do not represent all the types of communication problems and issues that may occur.

* * *

When the day nursing coordinator walked onto the busy thirty-eight bed medical and surgical patient unit at 7:00 a.m., she sensed tension beyond what usually prevailed. Her previous six years as a registered nurse had given her invaluable experience which had sharpened her intuition and judgment. Even before hearing the night nurse's report, this seasoned nurse sensed that the forty-four-year-old woman in the room near the nursing station was not stable. The patient had a long history of episodically severe asthma and now had staphylococcal pneumonia as an added diagnosis.

After thoroughly evaluating this patient, including reviewing her chart and lab work, the nursing coordinator believed the woman was in a precarious condition and would crash some time that morning. The night nurse reported that the patient's attending physician had come in at 6:00 a.m., decided she was stable, and wanted treatment continued as prescribed. The nursing coordinator was incredulous. She believed the patient needed more aggressive treatment and should be transferred to the intensive care unit (ICU).

She began with the usual protocol. She telephoned the physician and reviewed the patient's data adding her concerns. She requested the physician to return and reassess the patient. He adamantly refused and made it clear that he did not want this patient transferred to the ICU. Not satisfied, she continued to follow the protocol by turning to the next person in the chain of command. She sought advice from the nursing administrator who, in turn, contacted the chief of medicine. The stated consensus relayed back to her was that the patient should remain on the unit for further observation.

She could not let it rest. She firmly believed that this patient would crash within the next few hours. Either she had to obey her superiors or find a way to go around them. She knew she had to try to help this patient whom she felt was in dire need. If they wouldn't let this patient go to the ICU, maybe she could bring the ICU to her.

As nursing coordinator she telephoned the ICU coordinator and reviewed the situation to include stating that her request for this patient to go to the ICU had repeatedly been denied. Fortunately the eight bed ICU had only two patients who were almost ready to be transferred, so that unit was not busy. Because the ICU coordinator was available and realized that this situation seemed very serious, she immediately came over and examined the patient. She agreed that this patient was indeed unstable and did belong in the ICU. Since she was not authorized to admit patients to her unit, she sent an ICU nurse to help the nursing coordinator manage the patient on the medical surgical unit.

Both nurses immediately went to work. They put in another more effective intravenous line, put this critically ill woman on the usual intensive care monitoring and observation regime, and transferred her to an ICU stretcher. As expected, the patient crashed. Respiratory therapists who were now standing by intubated her within seconds of respiratory arrest. Now there was no question that this patient needed to be in the ICU. Because of the immediate and effective response to this patient's emergency, her transfer to the ICU was accomplished quickly and easily. The ICU physician was impressed with what the nurses had done. When the patient's physician heard about what happened and saw the nursing coordinator, he laughed somewhat sheepishly and muttered, "I guess you were right."

Even though the situation had been resolved and her accurate assessment acknowledged, the nursing coordinator felt some lingering frustration and anger. She was emotionally drained. She said it was very difficult to have been told to take no further action when she knew this patient had urgently needed more aggressive care.[2]

* * *

In *Safe Patients, Smart Hospitals* Dr. Peter Pronovost, anesthesiologist at Johns Hopkins Hospital, Baltimore, Maryland, related the following story. He remembered administering anesthesia to a patient who was being operated on for an abdominal hernia repair. About an hour and a half into the surgery her blood pressure dropped, her face turned red, she began wheezing, and she was having difficulty breathing. He knew these are classic symptoms of an allergic reaction, so he quickly reviewed her medications. She was not known to be allergic to any of them, so he suspected she was allergic to the surgeon's latex gloves. She'd had ten previous operations and allergic reactions to latex are common among patients who have had many surgeries where such gloves are used. When latex makes contact with the blood of allergic patients, these allergies can be severe. Within minutes these patients can skid into anaphylactic shock and die. Because he knew this he gave the patient epinephrine, the drug known to treat this condition. Her symptoms quickly disappeared.

Dr. Pronovost immediately told the surgeon he believed the patient was having a latex allergy reaction. He recommended to the surgeon that he change his gloves to a non-latex type, easy to do because the gloves are stocked in the operating room. The surgeon refused. "You're wrong. This can't be a latex allergy. We have been operating for an hour and a half and the patient didn't experience a reaction to latex during any of her previous procedures." Dr. Pronovost told him latex allergies can occur anytime, this patient had many previous surgeries, and the gloves had not come into contact with her blood until about an hour and a half into the surgery. That was why the reaction hadn't occurred earlier.

The patient's symptoms returned. Dr. Pronovost gave her another epinephrine dose. As before, her symptoms quicky responded. Now he was certain she had a latex allergy. Again he asked the surgeon to change his gloves. Again the surgeon refused. "There is no way this is a latex allergy and I am not changing my gloves." Dr. Pronovost pressed his case. "Let's think through this situation. If I'm wrong, then you will waste five minutes changing gloves. If you are wrong, the patient dies. Do you really think this risk-benefit ratio warrants you not changing your gloves?" "You're wrong, this is clearly not an allergic reaction," replied the surgeon, "so I'm not changing my gloves."

The resident standing next to Dr. Pronovost was ashen. The nurses were speechless. Dr. Pronovost stared at the surgeon. "How confident are you that this is not a latex allergy? What else do you think could be causing her problems?" The patient's blood pressure continued to drop dangerously. Her blood oxygen was low and she was wheezing again. Dr. Pronovost knew that if her exposure to latex was not stopped, she would die.

Because he had gained a reputation in the hospital as a respected leader in patient safety, Dr. Pronovost felt confident that the senior hospital leaders would not tolerate the surgeon's behavior and would support him. He could not stand there and let the patient die. He told the surgeon his refusal was unacceptable. He raised his voice and told one of the nurses to urgently page Dean Miller and Mr. Peterson. Ed Miller was then Dean of the

Johns Hopkins University School of Medicine. Ron Peterson was then President of Johns Hopkins Hospital. The nurse walked over to the phone, picked it up, and looked at Dr. Pronovost. "Page them now. This patient is having a latex allergy. I cannot let her die because we did not change gloves." As the nurse began to dial, the surgeon blurted out an expletive, dropped his gloves, and left to change them. Thanks to Dr. Pronovost the patient survived. Later tests confirmed that this patient was allergic to latex.

It was the first time Dr. Pronovost had worked with that surgeon. He believed that the two surgeons he usually worked with would most likely have changed their gloves if asked, because they had an established working relationship which usually supports better communication and teamwork. He added that many surgical teams who have not worked together might not trust or respect each other's judgment or skill.

Dr. Pronovost believes doctors are not the only ones to blame for poor communication, rather that "Poor communication and lousy teamwork are a problem in every level of health care, from administrative assistants to top executives. No person or department is immune to this problem."[3]

* * *

Because many hospital administrators and staff recognized the need to improve communication, by the early 2000s many hospitals had begun to put in writing their expected codes of behavior. At Maimonides Medical Center, Brooklyn, New York, every doctor had been required to sign a Code of Mutual Respect. Dr. Strongwater refused to sign. He considered it pathetic that you had to tell professionals how to behave. He related the following situation which changed his mind.

He was scheduled to perform a difficult, relatively new hip surgical procedure on a young woman. The operation would take about six hours, would require six pints of blood, and would rebuild her hip socket with her own bone. Because this patient had suffered bad reactions to banked blood, he agreed to use blood donated by her family. He understood that it had been stored.

Usually he requested the blood about two hours into the operation. Though he didn't remember why, soon after making the incision he told the nurse to call for the blood. He waited while he heard some rustling on the phone. He asked the nurse what was the problem. She said they were looking for the blood. He didn't feel he could wait. He packed the wound then got the head of the blood bank on the phone. He had already started a difficult operation, a nervous family was waiting, and he didn't have the blood he'd been told was stored.

The head of the blood bank told him there had been an emergency over the weekend, and they had used the family's blood for the emergency. His face turned red as he remembered how livid he felt. "If I could have reached through the phone and ripped her throat out, I would have," he said. "So here's your Code of Mutual Respect."

He composed himself and continued to say that he didn't care that they had used the blood. They saved someone's life. But that was the weekend and here it was Monday. "Why the hell didn't someone call me and say, 'Dr. Strongwater, the blood for your patient was used emergently'? Or say on Monday, 'Don't do the case, the blood's not available'?" He had to face the patient's mother and offer options. Either they could do the operation and use banked blood, or close the wound and schedule it another time. The mother told him to close the wound. Dr. Strongwater did the operation a month later.

He continued, "Here I am with all this experience, all this education, all this training, and look at this twit in the pipeline, the clerk who never made the call to notify me. You are relying on people with all levels of training, all levels of skill, all levels of commitment."

The hope was that the Code of Mutual Respect would prevent situations like this, that it would foster discussions, illuminate weak links, and improve the system. This situation led the hospital to tighten its procedures regarding segregating designated blood. Dr. Strongwater signed the Code because he came to believe that people should know that the Code did not just involve physicians and the operating rooms, the Code showed that the organization was serious about working conditions "across the board."[4]

* * *

In many hospitals the hierarchy is especially sharply defined in the operating rooms. The surgeons are the captains and do not always believe that their staff have skills or information they need. In "Good Doctors Spot Mistakes, Save Lives" a cardiac catheterization lab nurse told Dr. Richard Karl that she had tried to get a cardiologist to use the correct guide wire for an arterial catheter. The cardiologist ignored her information, perforated the patient's aorta, then told the patient's family that the subsequent need for emergency surgery was because of the nurse's mistake. "Do you think I'll ever try to help him again?" she asked.[5]

Dr. Peter Pronovost noted that many surgical teams do not know the names or roles of their colleagues even if they have worked together for years. He remembers seeing a nurse with tears in her eyes just after the surgeon had left the room. When he asked her what was the matter, she said, "I have worked for twenty years with him, I have bent over backward to make this place work and his life better, and he does not even know my name."[6]

* * *

Dr. Pronovost became intrigued by the similarities between aviation and medicine. Since checklists had improved airline safety, he was convinced checklists could improve patient safety. As an ICU physician at Johns Hopkins in 2000, he well knew about the problem of ICU central line catheter infections. Central line catheters are regularly used in intensive care. They allow for administering major drugs, such as epinephrine for cardiac arrest, directly to the heart. He estimated that nationally each year approximately 80,000 patients become infected and 30,000 to 60,000 patients die as a result of receiving central line catheters. He decided to try to reduce those infections by using a checklist.

After his team reviewed the 120 page guideline from the Centers for Disease Control and Prevention (CDC), talked with the nurses and physicians and observed how the central lines were being placed, the team settled on five key steps for their checklist. They distributed the checklist to the physicians. Then they asked the nurses to observe how well the physicians used it. Results were that the physicians were complying with the checklist only 38% of the time. That meant they were putting two out of three patients at risk of infection and death.

After doing the procedure himself and talking with his physician colleagues, he realized that they were often going to as many as eight different places to get the needed items. Some said they omitted steps because they didn't have time to hunt for what wasn't there. So, after asking the physicians what they needed, the team created a central line cart and assigned someone responsible for keeping the cart stocked. When the nurses observed the physicians who were now relying on the stocked cart, compliance jumped to 70%. This was certainly better, but not good enough. Dr. Pronovost wanted 100% compliance.

The team knew they needed independent monitors with authority to force the physicians to comply with the checklist. So Dr. Pronovost presented their plan to the staff. The nurses would monitor the physicians and make sure that they meticulously complied with the checklist. The nurses could demand any physician to immediately fix any error in following the steps. The traditional rigid hospital hierarchy reared its head. It was like World War III, said Dr. Pronovost. The physicians viewed the plan as eroding their power and authority. The nurses believed that if they followed the plan, they would get abuse and criticism from the physicians.

Dr. Pronovost had to convince the nurses of their crucial role in ensuring that the patients received the best possible care. He asked them how could they watch a doctor not follow the correct procedures when they were risking the patient's life in the process. He emphasized that he would guarantee they would be supported. They could page him if any of the physicians resisted. Also, each of the top executives gave the ICU teams the following message: "Page me or call my cell phone if the doctors don't comply with the checklist." To the doctors he said, "Let me make this really, really clear. Nurses will question you. If you make a mistake, you will go back and fix the problem the nurse identified . . . . I do not expect you to be perfect . . . . However, I do expect you to help create a system to ensure that patients always receive recommended therapies, that patients are not needlessly harmed." A year later the infection rates had dropped to almost zero.

Now that Dr. Pronovost had proof that a relevant enforced checklist could lower infections and improve patient safety in intensive care, he and his team expanded their efforts to include other hospital units. As before, it was the climate, the communication issues within and among various levels of the hospital hierarchy, that needed to be addressed. Too often in health care the staff most directly involved with patients are not asked for their ideas. Yet they are the ones most familiar with their work and their work environments. So Dr. Pronovost's team asked the unit members: "How do you think the next patient might be harmed? . . . What can you do to prevent it?"

Unit teams were established to continue to support the unit members. Each unit team included: a hospital executive, vice president or higher; a physician; a nurse; and associated staff, such as pharmacists or respiratory therapists. These teams went on patient rounds one hour each month. When staff accepted that communication regarding patient safety issues were expected, encouraged, and welcomed by the teams, they stated the problems. Given the composition of the teams, the teams were able to facilitate various needed solutions. Dr. Pronovost noted that executives had literally stopped him in the halls to proudly tell him that the rates of infection in their units were still low.

Dr. Pronovost believes that top executives joining with clinicians is a powerful tool for change. Their involvement on the units also supports staff morale, staff who often feel invisible and insignificant to the hospital administration. In Dr. Pronovost's words: "Executives uniquely hold the power to allocate resources, navigate politics, and increase awareness of issues across the entire hospital landscape."[7]

* * *

Dr. Pronovost has become known nationally for his program's results in reducing infections and improving patient safety at Johns Hopkins Hospital, and he is often a valued speaker. At a meeting in northern Michigan an older gray haired nurse from a small community hospital with a four bed ICU in the Upper Peninsula said to him, "I've got to tell you, Dr. Pronovost, you have changed my hospital. We were using your checklist and one of the senior doctors came in and didn't wash his hands. So I said, 'You've got to go back and fix this.' And he responded, 'What do you mean . . . . This is the way I put lines in.' I said, 'No, that is not the way you do it anymore. Dr. Pronovost says so, and if you don't go do it right now I am going to page him and tell him.' The doctor asked me, 'Who is Dr. Pronovost?' And I said, 'He is the ICU doctor from Johns Hopkins and I am going to page him if you don't do it the right way.' And he said, 'I have seen his research; he is doing great work. No, no, I don't want you to do that. I'll do it your way.'"[8]

* * *

Many hospitals in many states are now successfully using Dr. Pronovost's program. His program is crucial for patient safety in this day of superbugs that are not eradicated by available antibiotics. In the 2010 publication of his book *Safe Patients, Smart Hospitals*, Dr. Pronovost said "we are trying to implement this program across the United States, state by state, hospital by hospital."[9]

Speaking up to persons higher in a hierarchy can be difficult if the system doesn't support hearing questionable or contrary opinions. The airlines have well documented how lives can be saved or lost based on communication alone. Flight crews, which typically consist of a captain and one or more junior officers, are taught to speak up if they are aware of something amiss.[10]

* * *

Airline safety science, called Crew Resource Management (CRM), developed after a crash in 1978 near Portland, Oregon. Six miles short of the airport a United Airlines DC-8 ran out of fuel. The flight engineer knew the plane was running out of fuel, but didn't tell the captain until it was too late. Of the 189 passengers and crew, 10 died.[11]

In a severe snowstorm in January 1982, Air Florida Flight 90 crashed into the Fourteenth Street Bridge on the Potomac River in Washington, D.C. Seventy passengers, four crew members, and four motorists on the bridge died. Only five passengers survived when they were plucked from the icy Potomac River by firefighters. Errors began at the airport. Despite having not properly deiced the wings, the crew decided to proceed with takeoff. Airline safety officials considered the next error as even more serious. As the plane began lift off, the first officer did not believe they had enough power for a successful takeoff. He repeatedly voiced his concern while the captain continued to ignore his warnings. It was later confirmed that they had plenty of runway to abort takeoff.[12]

In the early to mid-2000s the pilots of Swiss Air Flight 111 disagreed about how to manage their emergency. Smoke was filling the plane and seeping into the cockpit. Protocol required going through a lengthy checklist. The captain insisted on staying with the checklist. The copilot repeatedly suggested steps that would have rapidly accomplished heading to the nearest airport for an emergency landing. The captain repeatedly rejected his copilot's advice and kept focusing on the checklist. A few minutes before the plane plunged into the ocean the captain told the copilot that he was in the middle of the checklist and did not want to be interrupted again. He wasn't. There was no more time. The plane crashed into the ocean, and all 230 passengers and crew died.[13]

* * *

In *The Checklist Manifesto* Dr. Atul Gawande, surgeon at the Brigham and Women's Hospital in Boston, Massachusetts, became interested in checklists as a way to reduce errors and improve patient safety. In January 2007 he joined the World Health Organization (WHO) sponsored convention of surgeons, anesthesiologists, nurses, safety experts, and patients from around the world to discuss what could be done to improve the safety and quality of surgical procedures around the world.

Their work, which included testing checklists in various countries, resulted in a final WHO safe surgery checklist which had been shown to improve patient safety in operating rooms. On January 14, 2009, WHO's safe surgery checklist was made public. By the end of 2009 about 10% of American hospitals and worldwide more than 2000 hospitals had either adopted the checklist or taken steps to implement it.[14]

Basic to the success of any checklist is how well the team members communicate with each other. In the usual surgical checklist there are three required pause points: before anesthesia, before the incision, and before the patient leaves the room. Before the operation begins the team members must introduce themselves by name and state their roles, the patient is identified, marking of the surgical site must be confirmed, and the surgeon describes the operation to include when potential problems might occur. The surgeon emphasizes to the team that any of them should speak up if they see any problems. The operation proceeds only when everyone confirms being ready.[15]

Researchers at various hospitals, including Johns Hopkins, noted that when nurses said their names and concerns before the operation proceeded, they were more likely to state problems and offer solutions. The Kaiser hospitals in southern California tested their checklist for six months in 3500 operations. Their staff rated the teamwork climate. Employee satisfaction rose 19%, and the rate of turnover for the operating room nurses dropped from 23% to 7%.[16]

Those not on the operating team, yet in the room, are expected to speak up. It is irrelevant where one is in the hospital hierarchy. Errors not caught may seriously compromise the effort toward safe patient care. The following story illustrates this point.

* * *

This situation occurred at Maimonides. Verification of the following had occurred: patient's name, the procedure, and the site. Just prior to the time of the incision, the presumed knee to be operated on was being prepped. Then someone asked loudly, "How come the knee being prepped isn't marked with a 'yes'?" The room became silent. A medical student, lowest on the professional hierarchy, had spoken. The "yes" was on the other knee. The final check had taken place too soon. The equipment had not been placed on the operating side. Everyone had assumed that the leg next to the equipment was the object of the surgery.[17]

* * *

Assumptions can indeed mislead. Unverified, incorrect assumptions can cause severe patient injury, even death. Dr. Gawande states, "Checklists supply a set of checks to ensure the stupid but critical stuff is not overlooked, and they supply another set of checks to ensure people talk and coordinate and accept responsibility." He adds, "There must always be room for judgment."[18] Though not so stated, checklists supported by honest communication from alert staff are designed to prevent incorrect, unverified assumptions, assumptions that could considerably compromise patient safety.

Hospital patients with their families and friends are also members of the hospital hierarchy. They, too, should speak up if they are aware of anything amiss. As told to me, one such patient, awake prior to cataract surgery, was alerted when the nurse who had been putting eye drops in the eye designated for surgery, put some in the other eye. "Hold on," he said, "that's not the eye that's being operated on." The nurse quickly moved to the other eye and put eye drops in there.

The airline industry was pressed to recognize and respond to the issue of airline safety long before the health industry began to tackle their issue of patient safety. In an airplane, if an urgent message is denied, the captain, the crew, and all the passengers may die. Airline disasters quickly become public knowledge. If hospital staff don't respond to the message that something is amiss, only the patient, not the staff, may die. The error may not be acknowledged or even known by others not directly involved.

The airline stories make the following points. In the first story the flight engineer doesn't tell the captain that the fuel is running out until it is too late. In the second story the captain ignores the first officer's warnings that there was not enough power for a successful takeoff in the raging snowstorm. In the third story the captain doggedly focuses on completing a checklist despite smoke filling the plane and seeping into the cockpit, even though his copilot repeatedly suggests steps that would rapidly accomplish heading to the nearest airport for an emergency landing. There is lateness in speaking up to the captain who is higher in the hierarchy, and there is lack of judgment and denial of urgency from the captains who repeatedly ignored their junior officers' warnings of impending disaster.

In the first hospital story from a medical surgical unit an experienced nursing coordinator makes the assessment that her critically ill patient needs intensive care. Her request that the attending physician return to re-evaluate the patient is denied by the physician and all the other professionals above her in the hierarchy, including the chief of medicine. She was told the patient should remain on the unit for further observation. She found this unacceptable. She had followed the designated protocol. Those involved had failed her. So she turned to the ICU's nursing coordinator, one on her same level in the hospital hierarchy. That coordinator sent an ICU nurse who agreed that this patient was critical. They did more for the patient. Soon thereafter, as expected, the patient crashed. Then admission to the ICU was allowed. Though the situation was finally resolved, the nursing coordinator was left with frustration and anger that she had been told to take no further action when she knew this patient needed more intensive care. The hierarchy failed her.

With a reputation in Johns Hopkins Hospital as a respected leader in patient safety, Dr. Pronovost is confident that if he pages the top of the hierarchy he will get the support he urgently needs for the surgeon to change his latex gloves when the patient was showing clear evidence of a latex allergy. He knows the patient will die if the surgeon continues to refuse changing his gloves. He tells the nurse to page the Dean of the Johns Hopkins School of Medicine and the President of Johns Hopkins Hospital. Before the page goes through, the surgeon swears and leaves to change his gloves. Taking steps to include the top brass resulted in resolving the desperate situation.

Dr Strongwater finally signed Maimonides' Code of Mutual Respect after being frustrated that a low level clerk hadn't informed him that the family's stored blood was no longer available for his patient. He had already begun the operation and learned this only when he called for the blood. The situation would have been considerably worse if he had followed his usual procedure of calling for the blood after about two hours into the operation. Because the patient previously had suffered severe reactions to banked blood, the operation was not continued per direction of the patient's mother. Dr. Strongwater hoped that the Code of Mutual Respect would result in improved communication "across the board."

Dr. Peter Pronovost and Dr. Atul Gawande have clearly shown that relevant, concise checklists used with good judgment lower rates of infection and thereby improve patient safety. However, for checklists to work, the staff need to own them, be part of them, contribute to them, and refine them as needed. Hospital hierarchies too often tend to be rigid in terms of authority and focus of responsibility within and between all levels.

When Dr. Pronovost and his team expanded their efforts to improve patient safety on hospital units other than the intensive care units, they leveled the usual hierarchy by including executives in unit teams so they would better understand and contribute to solving such issues. Problems were revealed and solutions found when the unit staff realized that these teams were sincere in wanting honest communication from them.

Executives may not realize how crucial their behavior with their staff is in setting the tone of their hospital system. Creative thinking and good morale occur only when all staff at all levels are treated as important members who are included in solving problems that inevitably occur. As stated in *Life and Death of a Mental Hospital*: "The greater freedom which members of an organization perceive themselves to have in coming to decisions, the more they will believe in the value of their activities."[19]

When staff are left out of important decisions that affect them, morale is lowered, they feel they don't count, there is a loss of creative ideas, and there tends to be more staff turnover. Staff who are dissatisfied with how they are treated in the system can add their feelings to an atmosphere that may adversely affect the quality of patient care and spill over into their communities, ultimately affecting the hospital's reputation.

These stories highlight the crucial importance of a free flowing supportive climate of communication within and between all levels in a hospital hierarchy as essential in promoting staff morale, in encouraging creative solutions from anyone in the system, in improving patient safety, and ultimately improving the quality of patient care.

17. Hierarchies

There were various feelings amongst the workers of some of Michigan's large automobile plants when their companies were down-sizing in the less than favorable economy of the early 2000s. At General Motors Kenneth Doolittle had supervised a team of assembly line workers. He spoke with pride about his job which had given him much self-esteem. "I loved all of it—the people, the work," he said. "I was in a position finally where people listened to me when I spoke. I wasn't just a Joe-Nobody. I contributed." However, after the plant where he worked was closed, and he was offered an assembly line job at another factory, he decided to leave and take a buy-out. "I did not want to start over, not after thirty-three-and-a-half years." He was fifty-four and felt it was too difficult to forfeit the higher rank he had worked many years to secure.

Leann Bies, at age forty-eight, had given twenty-nine years of service. She was an electrician at a Ford truck plant with only one year left to retirement. She accepted a buy-out that allowed her to stay home that last year and collect 85% of her pay, $65,000 annually. She'd also get $36,000 pension plus retiree health insurance. This package, plus Ford having paid tuition for her to earn a bachelor's degree in business leadership during her spare time, didn't change the fact that she was angry about "shoddy treatment" in her recent years there. She said the "management of this plant is very disrespectful." The plant produced a popular pick-up truck, and there was constant pressure to keep the line moving. "I came into this plant in 2003, and for two years they treated me as if I were dumber than a box of rocks." She added, "You get an attitude if you are treated that way. It is an important part of my decision to leave."[1]

* * *

Tod's is a successful multinational, multibillion dollar company in Italy that makes exquisite leather shoes and handbags. Diego Della Valle, its chairman, finds out if a new style of shoes is satisfactory by wearing them. If after a few days he doesn't like them they don't go into production. After wearing one such pair he stated, "I don't like the way they feel . . . . It's the part around the toes. It needs to be rounder." Tod's has refused to follow the trend of other Italian based multinational companies that moved production to cheaper places such as China. The company does not compromise on quality even when it may mean raising prices. Through the financial crisis from around 2007 through 2009 it was one of the few worldwide luxury companies that increased its sales and profits.

Tod's is a family business. Diego's younger brother, Andrea, manages operations. The company's headquarters are ten minutes from Diego's hilltop home, their family's retreat, in Casette d'Ete, Italy. In the light-filled campus, sketches are sent to a modeling room where about twenty employees print three dimensional casts for patterns. About fifty people make prototype shoes from leather cut manually along the blueprints. After Diego approves a model, it goes into production at a leather and sewing factory where the shoes are hand-stitched.

The family cares about their employees. Diego's father, at eighty-five, still makes rounds. Andrea spoke about his father. "He has a word for everyone, from the newest worker to the most senior manager." He sometimes speeds getting around by pedaling his bicycle around the halls. At their offices the brothers pointed to an old wooden table, the table that they, their father, and their grandfather had sat around, cutting leather and stitching shoes by hand. "It's there so we don't forget our roots," said Diego.[2]

* * *

Gore Associates, Newark, Delaware, is a multimillion dollar high-tech company with thousands of employees. The company makes water-resistant Gore-Tex fabric, Glide dental floss, insulating coatings for computer cables, and a variety of specialty cartridges, filter bags, and tubes for the automobile, semiconductor, pharmaceutical, and medical industries. Gore Associates has leveled the hierarchy. At Gore there are no titles. The business card of anyone who works there shows the person's name with "Associate" under that name. Headquarters are in a low slung unpretentious red brick building. The offices along a narrow corridor are small and plainly furnished. No one has a prestigious corner office. The corner areas tend to be conference rooms or free space.

Some years ago Wilbert "Bill" Gore, the late founder of the company, told an interviewer that "things get clumsy at a hundred and fifty." So the decision was made to stay with no more than 150 employees per plant. When the company expands, it continues to build same sized plants. There are fifteen plants within a twelve mile radius in Delaware and Maryland. As an example of how it stays within 150, their apparel business was divided into two groups. Boots, backpacks and hiking gear moved to another plant, while Gore-Tex uniforms for firefighters and soldiers remained in its own plant.

The advantage of this size group is that the process for designing, making, and marketing a given product is subject to the scrutiny of the same group. Peer pressure is powerful. People want to live up to what is expected of them. The manufacturing and sales people work together. The salesperson who wants to get a specific order taken care of can go to someone on the manufacturing team and work it out. People get to know each other's abilities and expertise. They come to know who can best solve a problem. Gore is a high technology company that relies on its ability to innovate and quickly respond to demanding and sophisticated customers. This model allows for new ideas and information to move easily within the organization.[3]

* * *

On July 10, 2006, two tons of the Big Dig Tunnel in Boston, Massachusetts, crashed, crushing and killing Milena Del Valle as she was her on her way through the tunnel in a car. It was reported that testing in 1999 revealed that the bolt and epoxy system that held the cement panel that killed Del Valle occasionally failed. Construction workers had questioned the safety of the system. Was anyone listening? Was shoddy work accepted as the norm?[4]

Dick Pereli wrote a letter to the *Boston Sunday Globe* about working with epoxy. He has been a boat builder for twenty-two years and works with epoxy every day. He said that what he had read about epoxy to secure concrete panels in the Big Dig sounded crazy. His small boat shop takes multiple steps to ensure that the epoxy they mix cures strong. Each batch is weighed and mixed. Then a small amount of pigment is added which gives them a visual cue. If the pigment is mixed, then they know the epoxy is mixed. After the resin cures in the boat, they check out the boat and the bucket of leftover resin to see that it is as hard and strong as it should be. He believes that in the case of such critical components as concrete ceilings, each batch of epoxy that was mixed should have had a little sample saved to test. "It is not expensive to do this. It is expensive not to do it," said Pereli.[5]

* * *

When Dr. Atul Gawande was thinking about checklists as a way to reduce errors and improve patient safety, he visited Joe Salvia, a structural engineer whose firm has provided the structural engineering for most of the major hospital buildings in Boston since the late 1960s, many of the hotels, office towers, and condominiums. His firm was also responsible for the structural rebuilding of Fenway Park, home of the Boston Red Sox baseball team. The McNamara/Salvia firm's specialty is designing and engineering large, complicated, high rise structures all over the country. Their tallest skyscraper is an eighty story tower in Miami. Dr. Gawande wanted to know how Salvia's firm works, especially how it builds in safety.

Salvia told him that "A building is like a body. It has a skin. It has a skeleton. It has a vascular system—the plumbing. It has a breathing system—the ventilation. It has a nervous system—the wiring." He said some sixteen different trades are often involved. He showed Dr. Gawande the construction plans for a four-hundred-foot-tall skyscraper he was building. The table of contents indicated that each trade had contributed its own section. All the contributions had to fit together, be precisely carried out, and in coordination. Salvia emphasized that failure in the construction business is not an option. When he designed his first shopping mall roof he quickly understood there was no margin for error. Many people could die if his roof collapsed under the weight of snow.

Salvia took Dr. Gawande to one of the construction sites where he and his team were building a sprawling thirty-two-story, 700,000 square foot office and apartment complex with a two acre footprint. There, in the field office, he met Finn O'Sullivan, project executive. On the walls of the main conference room hung sheets of butcher-block-size printouts of checklists. On one wall was the construction schedule: a line-by-line, day-by-day listing of every building task, in what order, and when it needed to be accomplished. The schedule involved multiple sheets with color coding. Red items highlighted critical steps that had to be done before other steps could proceed. As each task was completed a job supervisor reported to O'Sullivan, who put a check mark in the computer scheduling program and posted a new printout showing the phase of work to be accomplished each week.

Bernie Rouillard, Salvia's lead structural engineer, took Dr. Gawande on a tour. The building was being built in layers. Dr. Gawande looked at the bare metal trusses that had been put in the ceiling to support the next floor being built. Rouillard told him the fireproofers would come next. Dr. Gawande was surprised. "You have to fireproof metal?" The answer was a resounding yes. Rouillard told him that metal in a fire can plasticize, lose its stiffness, then bend like spaghetti. Rouilland explained that this was why the World Trade Center buildings collapsed. Dr. Gawande continued the tour, astounded at the complex and intricate process that was taking place.

From recent rain, on each of the open floors large amounts of water had pooled against the walls of the inner concrete core making the floors seem tilted. Rouillard believed that since the outer steel frame had not been loaded with its weight, the immense weight of the concrete core on the soil underneath probably had caused the core to settle sooner than anticipated. Rouillard believed that once the steel frame was loaded with another eighteen stories yet to be built, the floor would level out. He acknowledged that variances do occur.

Salvia had told Dr. Gawande that in medieval and much of modern times buildings had been built by Master Builders who designed, engineered, and oversaw construction from start to finish. But now there could be many specialists involved. To Dr. Gawande, this sounded similar to the way medical care had evolved: a physician who used to make all the decisions, now many specialists may become involved. He wondered how these builders dealt with their unexpected complications.

Back at the field office Dr. Gawande asked O'Sullivan what they do when problems arise. O'Sullivan told him that they do not trust only one set of checklists to make sure that simple steps are not missed, they also have another set to make sure that everyone talks through and resolves conceivable, unexpected problems. It is assumed that anything can go wrong, anything can get missed. It is also believed that if you get the right people together and they talk together as a team, serious problems can be identified and averted. The original schedule included the various experts who must talk with each other as the trades are involved. When a problem occurs, persons relevant to solving the problem get together as a team and sort it out.

In 1978, a year after the Citicorp building opened, a Princeton engineering student's question led to the discovery that there had been a change in the building plan that had bypassed a checkpoint. Because it was cheaper and less labor intensive, Bethlehem Steel had switched to bolted joints instead of the welded joints specified in the original plan. Calculations regarding the resulting difference in joint strength were not reviewed by a specialist. This change led to a serious flaw, because it meant that the building would not withstand seventy-mile-an-hour winds which occur at least once every fifty-five years in New York City. If that happened the joints would fail. Starting on the thirtieth floor the building would collapse. The tower was already occupied. The owners and city officials were informed. That summer, as Hurricane Ella headed toward the city, an emergency crew secretly worked at night to weld two-inch thick steel plates around the two hundred critical bolts which secured the building.

By using checklists which include experts talking together as a team to anticipate problems, then working through changes and problems as they occur, the construction industry has a reputation for constructing safe buildings including skyscrapers. Finn O'Sullivan succinctly made this same point to Dr. Gawande when he said, "The biggest cause of serious error in this business is a failure of communication."[6]

* * *

Ingrid Bengis-Palei founded Ingrid Bengis Seafood in Stonington, Deer Isle, Maine in 1985. A native of New York City, Ingrid fell in love with Stonington with its small town resident population after only a day's visit with her father in the 1960s. In 1970 she bought a $2,000 house without running water. Somewhere in the 1980s on a trip to New York City she noticed that an epicurean market was charging a fortune for chanterelle mushrooms which were plentiful in the Deer Isle spruce forests, and which she had been picking for herself. She called the shop's buyer who agreed to purchase any chanterelles she could gather. Midway into the mushroom season the buyer told her he needed 100 pounds of lobster. She procured them, put them in her truck, and shipped them from the airport in Bangor, Maine. Thus began Ingrid Bengis Seafood whose cedar-shingled barn now houses the packing and shipping department.

Ingrid collects orders for a variety of seafood including oysters, crab, clams, mussels, halibut, scallops, and lobsters, all of which have to be acquired, iced, packed, and shipped usually the same day. Ingrid has a close relationship with everyone from the fishermen to the buyers, many of whom are high ranking chefs who prepare meals for their high-end customers. She will not deal with chefs who are not interested in getting to know the people who provide their seafood. One sous chef wouldn't listen to her stories about them. "He told me he was just trying to buy lobsters," said Ingrid. "I told him, 'Then buy from someone else.'" Ingrid made clear her feelings when she said, "A lobster is not just something on your plate; it's someone's life. Every other year someone dies on the water. I have tremendous respect for these people."

When Ingrid began her company a single container of crabmeat might contain a mixture of any species that scurried into lobster traps. Ingrid realized that the meat of one variety, locally called picket toe, was sweeter and milder than the others, so she refused to buy any other type. Later the owner of the premium seafood distributor Browne Trading in Portland, Maine, popularized the name peekytoe, and chefs clamored to have it on their menus.

Most commercial crabmeat is packed by machine resulting in containers that include shards of shell and flakes of cartilage. A good crab picker picks crab clean, but can produce only ten to fifteen pounds a day. Ingrid is as concerned about those who pick the crab as she is about those who fish for it. Her crab pickers mark their containers so chefs know the source of their peekytoe. When she stopped to talk with crab pickers Sonia Bunt, Sonia's daughter, April, and Sonia's mother, she asked April about her college plans and why it was that she was considering taking courses online rather than attending a college elsewhere. Later Ingrid learned that Sonia had just been diagnosed with leukemia and was to be hospitalized for five weeks of treatment. Ingrid asked Sonia's husband if there was anything she could do. "Just keep buying our crab meat, Ingrid," he said as his voice cracked. April and her grandmother were planning to continue the work.

As Ingrid changed the crab market, she changed the scallop market. She never liked scallops brought in by large commercial draggers that stay out a week or more and haul huge nets over the sea floor. She started buying from small day boats or scuba divers who pluck scallops one by one off the bottom by hand. Chefs say they twitch when cut into because they are so fresh. By the mid-1990s "divers scallops" became the rage.

Metal canisters of scallops are labeled with the name of the person who harvested them. Every halibut comes with a tag with the name of the fisherman who caught it. Muller, one of her buyers, said a cod used to be just a cod. But when buying from Ingrid, she'd say, "Paul is on his way in with two 25-pounders." Or if Muller told her that "those were really good lobsters." She'd say, "Andy caught them." One of her crab pickers left a message that she could not deliver the order until the next day, which, Ingrid said, had left her screwed for the day. Ingrid knew this woman was having problems from a recent divorce. She also knew she would talk the chefs into changing their menus.

If not beloved by everyone, Ingrid Bengis-Palei is respected. She's just as forthright with her suppliers about how they should run their businesses including what she specifically wants relative to the quality of their seafood, as she is with the chefs in encouraging them to identify those who caught, dived for, or processed her seafood. Over the years top chefs have visited Deer Isle to pay homage to Ingrid's suppliers. Likewise do the suppliers honor her. "I know all about Ingrid and her fussiness, and it's a good thing," said Virginia Olsen, who sells clams to her. "She keeps my name on the product and is getting it out to a very high-end market. I don't know anyone who can promote our seafood as well as she does."[7]

* * *

At the automobile plant Ken spoke with pride about his job which had given him much self-esteem. "I wasn't just a Joe-Nobody.

I contributed." When his plant closed he took a buy-out because he felt it too difficult to forfeit the higher rank he had worked many years to secure. Leann accepted a buy-out at her automobile plant because she was angry about being treated as if she were "dumber than a box of rocks." Both are telling us how important it is to be treated with respect. Joe said his job had given him much self-esteem. Leann felt the way she had been treated could give anyone an attitude. How a hierarchy treats its employees is shown by what employees say about working there, and, when given a choice to stay or leave, can considerably influence that decision.

Tod's is a family business and a hierarchy that treats its employees with respect. Diego Della Valle, its chairman, has an eighty-five-year-old father who still makes rounds with a word for everyone from the newest worker to the most senior member. The old wooden table that their grandfather, father, and the sons had sat around, cutting leather and stitching shoes by hand is still there "so we don't forget our roots," said Diego.

Gore Associates has leveled its hierarchy. Everyone is called an Associate. To foster free flowing communication and creative ideas, no plant has more than one hundred fifty employees. Manufacturing and sales people are together. A plant this size allows for the possibility for manufacturing and sales people to learn about each other's abilities and expertise so they can work together and innovate, as needed, for the benefit of the customer.

Construction workers on the Big Dig Tunnel in Boston had questioned the safety of the bolt and epoxy system that held the cement panel that crashed onto a car killing Melina Del Valle. Later a letter to the *Boston Sunday Globe* from someone experienced in using epoxy tells us how inexpensive and easy it is to assure that epoxy is safe.

Dr. Atul Gawande was considering checklists as a way to reduce errors and improve patient safety in health care. He went to a construction firm that builds major hospital buildings and large, complicated high rise structures. He learned that those involved are meticulous with each step in the designing and building process. There is a hierarchy which includes various levels of authority and expertise. However, everyone along the way is responsible for ensuring safety. It is assumed that anything can go wrong, anything can get missed. They have checklists to make sure that simple steps are not missed. They have another set to make sure that everyone talks through and resolves conceivable, unexpected problems. They believe that any serious problems can be identified, or if they occur, can be resolved if the right people get together and talk together as a team. This is a responsible, supportive hierarchy at its best. Like the airline industry, they know one minor problem can have a domino effect and could result in many lives injured or lost.

Ingrid Bengis-Palei understands the importance of treating people with respect. It is clear that she cares about the folks with whom she is involved. The fishing industry has a hierarchy of sorts. The fishermen are on the bottom rung. No so with Ingrid. She makes sure that her buyers, usually the chefs, know who have procured and processed the seafood. She won't sell to anyone who doesn't care about her people. Another hierarchy at its best. Her people are as important to her as is the product she sells.

Hierarchies are designed according to levels of authority and ability. How persons in hierarchies view their responsibilities in relation to their services or products cannot be separate from how they treat the people within their hierarchies if they truly believe that quality and safety are important.

18. The Milieu in Health Care

The atmosphere of a health care milieu is influenced by the physical environment and by the people who are there. How the atmosphere affects us as patients is determined by the thoughts and emotions it arouses in us, as well as the thoughts and emotions we bring to it. Though we are a captive audience, to whatever degree we are able, we can decide how much we will let it influence us. But when our resources are low, the milieu can have its greatest influence.

* * *

In December of her seventy-third year, the author May Sarton was diagnosed with congestive heart failure caused by a fibrillating heart. Her physician put her on various medications hoping to have her heartbeat return to normal. The following February she awoke in the middle of the night with a numb left arm, terrified feelings, and a brief hospitalization where a computed axial tomography (CAT) scan revealed a small brain hemorrhage. She was told she had suffered a mild stroke. Now with depression and the enormous effort to write even one line, she stated that the absence of psychic energy was staggering.

In May she awoke feeling unable to breathe. She thought she was suffocating. She returned to her local hospital and improved only after much fluid was removed from one of her lungs. In writing about that hospitalization she mentioned what had helped sustain her. "From my window I look beyond the parking lot to a beautiful line of trees against the sky. Two are just swelling into leaf, horizontal branches in wide curves. They are my food, my peace, these days. How could we live without trees?"

By the end of June she was scheduled for a cardioversion, a procedure that involves using an electric shock to return a fibrillating heart to a normal rhythm. For a half hour or more before the procedure she felt tense as she was lying on the narrow bed in Intensive Care. So she decided to invent a game of visualizing. She thought she'd visualize a flower, but finally focused on a picture of her beloved cat's face. When she realized his face looked like a crumpled pansy she found herself smiling. She said she "felt pleased to have invented a device against nervous tension."

In two different hospitalizations she turned to books. In June at her local hospital she finished the biography of Helen Waddell and said, "I'm glad I had it with me." In August she was at the Massachusetts General Hospital in Boston, Massachusetts, for an operation to readjust her heartbeat to allow for a cardiac pacemaker. Their evaluation revealed that her heart was weaker than had been expected, so the operation and pacemaker were cancelled. A friend had brought her *The Hospice Movement* by Sandol Stoddard. Referring to that hospitalization May said, "The thing that saved me that last night was reading the Hospice book . . . . It took me right out of self pity and ugly surroundings to pure love."[1]

* * *

I was immersed in my book. Suddenly it seemed eerily quiet. I looked up. The waiting room of my periodontist's office was empty. I saw no staff behind the window of the admitting office. No one in sight. The door to the corridor where the various offices were was closed. Was everyone gone? Did they forget me? The door opened. A staff member motioned for me to follow her.

I was there for three dental implants. I had insisted having all done the same day so I wouldn't have to keep traveling the two hour round trip for separate procedures. Since it was early afternoon and the waiting room had emptied, I realized it would probably be a long afternoon.

About as soon as I was tipped back in the chair, I noticed just above me a hummingbird mobile. A few birds were moving in a slight breeze. My periodontist asked if I were okay. I nodded and refocused on the birds. He went to work. I barely noticed what he and his assistant were doing, or felt anything after the needle pricks to numb the area. I decided to take the birds to Florida and watch them fly north through all the eastern states until they reached us in central New Hampshire. I had spent some time in Florida, various times at conferences in some of the other states, knew the sights of Washington, D.C., and was very familiar with eastern areas of all the New England states. I imagined the birds stopping at various flowers as they made their way north.

A male voice intruded. It was my periodontist asking if I were okay. My birds were now roaming around the southern Connecticut shoreline. I didn't want to lose them, so I quickly put up my fingers in an okay sign and returned to the birds. The procedure wasn't finished by the time they reached New Hampshire, so I returned them to Cape Cod in Massachusetts. Before the birds had returned, the periodontist said we were done. I almost felt reluctant to leave them until they were back with us. The procedure had taken two to three hours, but I had been oblivious to the length of time. I realized the hours had flown by only when I walked through the empty waiting room and out into the late afternoon sun.

* * *

Janice Carpenter was a librarian in Los Angeles, California. When she was forty-one she was diagnosed with amyotrophic lateral sclerosis, otherwise known as Lou Gehrig's disease. She well knew what she was facing. Deterioration proceeds relentlessly over the next three to five years, the usual life span of those with this disease. Janice continued on much longer than expected, about eleven years, during which time she became quadriplegic with flexion contractures at every joint. She was fed through a tube that had been inserted directly into her stomach. She occupied only a very small space in her bed. Because her facial muscles were paralyzed she was unable to talk, so an engineer connected her facial muscles to a computer to allow her to communicate.

With her permission her neurologist brought groups of senior medical students to a conference room to visit with her. The neurologist would ask them if they would want to be kept alive if they were in her condition. But before they could answer, a student would be encouraged to ask Janice how she felt about being kept going day after day in that state. They never turned their eyes away from the computer as she laboriously responded in what seemed an endless amount of time. Her answer was always the same. "My life may look dehumanized and infantilized, and it is. But I have a window next to my bed, and every morning I watch the sun rise, and hear the birds sing. And for me, that is a gift. That is why, yes, I want to live."[2]

* * *

In 1976 two scientists studied the perception of control among residents aged sixty-five to ninety at Arden House, a nursing home in Connecticut. The nursing home's social coordinator held separate meetings for the residents of two different floors.

He gave a plant to each resident at the first floor meeting. He told those residents that the nurses would take care of their plants for them. He said that there would be a movie on Thursdays and Fridays and they would be scheduled to see the movie on one of those days. He reassured them that they were permitted to visit people on other floors and involve themselves in different activities of their choosing, such as reading, watching television, listening to the radio. "We feel it is our responsibility to make this a home you can be proud of and happy in, and we want to do all we can to help you." The message was that these residents were allowed to do some things, but their well-being was the responsibility of the competent staff.

In the residents' meeting on the other floor the social coordinator let each resident choose which plant he or she wanted, and told them it was their responsibility to take care of their own plants. He told them they could choose whether to watch the weekly movie on Thursday or Friday, and reminded them about the many ways they could choose to spend their time, such as visiting with other residents, reading, listening to the radio, watching television. He emphasized that it was their responsibility to make their home a happy place. "It's your life," he said. "You can make of it whatever you want."

The staff treated the residents on the two floors in the same way and gave them the same amount of attention. Though the amount of control given each group was not considerably different, comparing the two groups at the end of three weeks showed some interesting results. The residents who were given more choice were more alert and happier. They interacted more with other residents and staff. Over 90% had improved physical health and six months later were less likely to have died. There was deterioration of physical health for over 70% of the group given less choice. And, compared with the group given more choice, they interacted less with the other residents and staff.[3]

* * *

The nurse manager of a geriatric psychiatry unit was making rounds one evening when she heard a patient crying in a little girl's voice. The patient was pleading for her mother and for her doll. Because she had been physically and verbally aggressive, which included being uncooperative when given care, she had been admitted from a nursing home. The nurse manager asked a mental health aide to take a pillowcase and make her a doll.

The patient hugged the doll as soon as she received it. She smiled and became calmer. She was more cooperative during procedures, tests, and when staff gave her care. She began to interact better with both staff and peers, and her sleep improved. Because these positive results continued, she was discharged shortly thereafter.[4]

* * *

In *Lost in America* Sherwin B. Nuland, M.D., described his and his family's emotional turmoil throughout his mother's failing health and subsequent death when he was a young boy. His mother was taken care of at home, and died there a week after his eleventh birthday. Esther, a nurse in her late twenties, came daily for a ten hour shift to care for her. He described Esther's influence: "It may have been her quiet cheerfulness, or the way she handled every small crisis with sweet-tempered imperturbability, but whatever the reason, she brought a new atmosphere . . . . Esther's efficient calm and self-assurance generated an unaccustomed air of order and control, which subtly transformed the mood of every one of us, even in the face of the unfolding events . . . . Her effect was felt even when she was not physically among us."[5]

* * *

During a life threatening illness Angelica Thieriot was admitted to a hospital with bare white walls. There was excessive noise, visiting was limited, and nightly disturbances were inevitable. She was not given adequate access to information about her condition or her treatment. She found the atmosphere impersonal and alienating. About half way through her hospitalization two nurses came into her room and called her by name. She remembers this as the first time any staff had addressed her directly. She felt encouraged and wanted to work with them toward getting better. She survived the illness and credits her ultimate healing to these two nurses.

Because of that experience Angelica Thieriot envisioned a hospital where caring, kindness, and respect are considered as crucial to patient healing as is technical skill. She brought together a group of physicians, hospital administrators, patients, writers, and architects. They founded the Planetree organization from their vision that hospitals would be designed with patient centered care as the central goal, rather than the convenience of practitioners being the central goal. The name Planetree was chosen because it was the type of tree under which Hippocrates, the father of medicine, sat and taught. His view was considered holistic because he considered patients from the multiple perspectives of body, mind, and spirit.

The first Planetree model was a thirteen bed medical surgical unit which opened in 1985 at San Francisco's Pacific Presbyterian Medical Center. The walls had bright colors and cheerful artwork. The staff kitchenette became available to patients, their families, and their visitors. A patient resource room was made available to patients and their families. The patients were invited to review their medical records and discuss them with staff. The patients became more actively involved in their treatment, and the staff became satisfied with this new model of care. These results were documented in a study by the University of Washington which led to the development of other model sites in New York, Oregon, and California during the late 1980s and early 1990s. Architects, professionals, and executives of health care facilities began to visit and study the hospitals with the Planetree model units. In another ten to fifteen years the Plantree organization encompassed a network of member sites throughout the United States, Canada, and Europe, all of which adhered to the Plantree ideals.[6]

* * *

My husband's sister, Charmian, had just passed her eightieth birthday when it was obvious that the leukemia was changing her life. She could care for herself and her three dogs, but she was in more and more pain, progressively more and more tired, and was doing less around her house and yard. She'd had a few admissions to her regional hospital, and one to the Maine Medical Center in Portland, Maine. She'd had various transfusions, and both her physician and oncologist had been working with her regarding managing her pain, but there was nothing else known that would improve her situation. She was given optimal opportunity to ask questions and receive relevant information. As a retired physician well informed about her circumstances, she well understood her situation. When she telephoned and told her brother, David, that she was being transferred to Gosnell House, Hospice of Southern Maine, we realized that she had turned a corner.

David and Charmian were not only brother and sister, they had a close friendship. I had known both of them since we were children because we played together as next door neighbors. So when I returned home and married David, the boy next door, Charmian came back into my life. Because of our health care careers we had many lively discussions. We had also become close, and I, as well as David, felt sadness in realizing that she might not be with us much longer. However, because we were familiar with the hospice concept for terminally ill patients, we were somewhat comforted that she would be in an atmosphere more like a home than a hospital, and that she would be given the best possible physical, emotional, and spiritual support by competent staff.

We easily found Gosnell House in its residential district in Scarborough, Maine. As we first walked in the door in the middle of the V-shaped wings we saw a living room with a fireplace, a kitchen and dining room, a foyer with a window seat, and signs indicating rest rooms. The walls had soothing colors. As we passed the kitchen a man who was cooking asked if he could get us coffee or anything else. We declined but thanked him. The person at the main desk welcomed us, told us where Charmian's room was, and that she'd have her nurse come see us. Within minutes I asked her nurse whether medications had been able to lessen her pain, and, basically, how was she doing. Her nurse understood that as a licensed health care professional I wanted specific detail, which she easily supplied. David and I were encouraged and relieved that Charmian was doing well under the circumstances, and that she was getting excellent care.

Charmian's room was spacious. She looked comfortable in a roomy bed that had a view of trees where a few birds were flying from limb to limb. We declined the offer of staying the night on a couch that could be made into a double bed. For two weeks we visited her almost daily. Except for her last few days she was able to reminisce with us, as old friends will. Later I wrote the Gosnell staff a note complimenting them for their care and their facilities. I told them they were well living up to the hospice concept with which I was familiar because I knew Florence Wald who is credited with bringing the hospice movement to the United States from England, and she had given me a tour of the hospice house in Branford, Connecticut.

* * *

Especially when we are patients we need to feel we have some control, and we need to feel comforted. Since we are part of the milieu, to whatever degree we are able, we can contribute to how it affects us. We may need to find diversions from the situation itself. Seeing the natural world including trees, birds, plants, and the sky can be very soothing, if available, and if we allow ourselves to tune into it. We can use our imaginations to visualize anything that interests us, and we can read. Other possible diversions will vary according to the situation and the people involved.

May Sarton and Janice Carpenter looked through their windows to see the sky, the sun, trees, or birds, and were sustained. I saw the hummingbirds in the mobile in my periodontist's office moving in the slight office breeze. With my imagination I joined their world and was oblivious to the procedure of three implants during a long afternoon. As I used my imagination for visualization of the hummingbird trip, May Sarton used visualization in thinking about her cat. She was pleased to have turned to visualization as a way to reduce her nervous tension.

The physical health of the residents of Arden House improved when they were responsible for their own plants and could choose which night they saw the movie as compared with those whose plants were taken care of by the staff, and told which night to see the movie. Compared with the last group, those in the first group were also more alert and happier.

In two different hospitalizations May Sarton mentioned reading books. I read mine in the periodontist's waiting room. I always take a book to any health care appointment, because I never know how long I may have to wait.

The geriatric patient in the psychiatric unit who had been admitted because of physical and verbal aggression was unable to soothe herself. She needed someone in the milieu to help her find a way to become calm. When the nurse manager heard her cry for her mother and her doll, the nurse manager knew she could not supply her mother, but she could supply a doll. It was stunning to see the change in this patient once she received a doll she could cuddle. She not only settled down and accepted the staff's care, she interacted better, her sleep improved, and she was shortly thereafter discharged.

The nurse who saw the Nuland family through the death of Sherwin's mother brought a sense of control and calmness into their apartment. Her manner, including her self-assurance, was such a steadying influence that the mood of the family remained transformed even when she was not physically there.

Angelica Thieriot credited two nurses for getting her through her life threatening illness. Her hospitalization in a noisy, impersonal environment with many disturbances had felt alienating. When these two nurses came in, the first staff to directly address her and call her by name, she felt encouraged to get better and to work with them. Her group that later founded the Planetree organization made clear their vision. Hospitals should be designed with patient centered care as the central goal. Caring, kindness, and respect must be recognized as just as crucial to patient healing as is technical skill. Because hospice environments are patient centered, Charmian, my sister-in-law, was fortunate to be in a quintessential hospice house.

So how is it that I knew Florence Wald, pioneer of the United States hospice movement? From 1959 to 1966 Florence Wald was Dean of the Yale University School of Nursing, New Haven, Connecticut. Prior to her years as dean she had been a faculty member there. I was a student in the Master of Nursing (M.N.) Program from 1955 to 1958 when Ida Orlando was doing her research on nurse-patient communications and continually telling us to "never assume." From 1959 to 1961 I majored in psychiatric-mental health nursing as a student in the Master of Science in Nursing (M.S.N.) Program under Ida Orlando during Florence's early years as dean. In 1961 I was hired by Florence to join the faculty where I remained through her deanship and some years beyond. Ida left for the Boston area in 1961 when she married Bob Pelletier. So the three of us knew each other and well knew what we felt was important as nurses in patient care. Patients with their needs must be the focus of care.

Florence's interest in hospice began in 1963 when she heard a lecture by Dame Cicely Saunders, a British physician who was planning to open the world's first hospice in Sydenham, south of London, England. Dr. Saunders' hospice, St. Christopher's, opened in 1967. Florence went to St. Christopher's to learn more about hospice, then returned to New Haven where she and others worked tirelessly to bring the hospice concept to the New Haven area. In November 1971, New Haven Hospice was incorporated as a non-profit corporation in Connecticut. I recall that hospice home visits became more and more available, because I supervised some of our Yale School of Nursing students who were making those visits.

In 1974 the New Haven Hospice board of directors bought land for a hospice house in Branford, about fifteen minutes by car from New Haven. Adequate finances and acceptance by the community took time, so it was some years more before the Connecticut Hospice House was ready for patients and their families. By the early 1980s Florence gave me a tour. As expected it was a warm, welcoming environment for patients and their visitors. Large windows afforded views of the sky, trees, birds, and the grounds. Because there was a nursery nearby, children were playing outside. The tour included all that I have previously described about the Gosnell House in Maine. Florence well understood how pleased I was with their success and grateful for her tour.

About a year or so before Ida Orlando's death in November 2007, Florence went to Massachusetts to see Ida. Knowing that Ida and I were close friends, Florence telephoned me about the visit. In that conversation I asked if she remembered that when she left as dean from the Yale School of Nursing she had left a plant on the desk of each of her faculty. She was quiet only a moment, then said, "Oh yes, I remember." I told her that my plant is now three plants. The largest brightens the living room. The smaller ones are in my office and waiting room. She said she knew I had a psychotherapy practice. Then she asked, "So what was the plant I gave you?" "I haven't the foggiest idea. I can't find it anywhere. Knowing how important plants have always been to you and hospice, I just call it Florence's plant," I replied. She laughed as we ended on that pleasant note.

Florence died in November 2008, leaving an extraordinary legacy. The hospice concept has exploded across the country. As I write this chapter I am between visiting houses in my area on the 24th Annual Hospice Home and Garden Tour to which huge numbers of tickets were sold in support of raising monies for our regional Hospice. Three of my relatives have used their services, and their families feel they could not have managed home care without the pain management, the team of specialists, and the ever continuing warm, caring support.[7]

In recognition of the importance of the milieu in health care, professionals involved in health care architecture and design are now joining with health care professionals and community members to develop patient centered health care environments to better respond to unique patient needs.[8] Such environments, however, are only as good as the communication therein. As patients, when we are able, as some of these stories have shown, we can help ourselves through our situations. When our resources are low, we need more assistance from others who are there. As Orlando discovered, it's crucial for staff to be sure they know what the patient needs before they take action to resolve those needs. Only then can the milieu be an optimal health care environment that responds well to unique patient needs.

19. Recognizing Assumptions

When we make an assumption we take something for granted. We accept it as fact. We learn assumptions early in our lives. They tell us what to believe, what to expect, or how to behave. Correct assumptions can simplify our lives. However, as many of the stories have shown, incorrect assumptions may lead us into various situations which can range from minor misunderstandings to disastrous outcomes. We may not always know when others make assumptions about us, but we can make a conscious effort to recognize our assumptions.

Orlando believed we behave automatically when we act on unrecognized assumptions, deliberatively when we recognize and verify our assumptions. The following story with its analysis illustrates this distinction.

* * *

Morley and Millie were brother and sister in their sixties. They had inherited their Vermont homestead from their parents who had died some fifteen years ago. Because neither had married nor wished to move, and their parents counted on them to help with chores, they had always lived at the McKerin Farm. After their parents died they had the option to sell their twenty acres to a developer. That was out of the question. They loved the farm with its apple orchids, pumpkin and produce gardens, their two working horses, the chickens, and a couple geese that followed them around. They had a seasonal produce stand that was popular in the area. With Markus, their German Shepherd, Morley and Millie would keep the McKerin Farm as long as they were able.

It was a brisk fall morning when Millie noticed that there was a frayed area in an electric wire that was attached to the house from the top of the pole across the driveway about fifty feet from the house. The frayed area was near the house and very noticeable against the blue sky. She was on her way to the kitchen door with eggs she had gathered from their chickens. Morley was out in the barn, but she expected he'd soon be back. When he came in she told him about the wire. He immediately followed her outside. Both were surprised that there were a few places where the wire was frayed. They had not had any symptoms that hinted of an electrical problem. She agreed to telephone their area electric company to come evaluate the situation to see what should be done.

When she called the electric company a woman answered. Millie explained that she was at the McKerin Farm, and she was concerned about frayed areas in a wire coming from the pole across the driveway to the house. The woman was pleasant and asked if the frayed wire was at the pole. "No," said Millie, "the frayed areas are near the house." The woman repeated the message which assured Millie that she clearly understood the problem. Though the McKerin Farm was a few miles from the electric company, the woman said she knew where the farm was and that an electric lineman would be there the next morning.

Millie and Morley were eating breakfast early the next morning when Millie just happened to look out the breakfast nook window and see a man in yellow coveralls, jacket, and hard hat walking briskly down the driveway. The driveway snaked down a hill around some large maples for about a tenth of a mile to the main road. She could see a yellow truck with blinking lights at the bottom of the driveway. "Morley, the lineman is here, but he's walking down the driveway! I'm going to catch up with him and find out what's going on!" She abruptly got up, rushed out the kitchen door, and ran down the driveway. She was almost breathless when she reached the truck at the bottom of the hill.

The lineman was sitting high up in the passenger side of his huge truck and was concentrating while writing something down. Though the truck door was opened, he didn't see Millie, so she banged on the metal door with her fist. He looked down at her. Because it was very windy she realized he wouldn't hear her, so she motioned him down. He put aside his writing, climbed down from the truck, and stood in front of her. He immediately said that the short capped wire hanging down from the pole was not an electric wire. "It's an old cable television wire and is not a problem." "I know that," she quickly responded. "That is not what concerns us. Didn't you see the frayed areas on one of the wires?" He didn't answer. "Please come and look." She turned and motioned for him to follow. He hesitated, then started walking with her up the long driveway. In conversation he acknowledged that he had planned to leave and report back to the office.

By the time they reached the top of the driveway Morley was outside looking at the wiring. Both he and Millie pointed to various places where the wire was frayed. The lineman seemed surprised and admitted he hadn't seen any frayed wire. He scrutinized the wire from the house to the pole and noticed more frayed areas than either Millie or Morley had seen. Millie asked him why he hadn't driven his truck up the driveway. Though he could now see that there was plenty of room, he said he hadn't known there would be room to turn around. He told Morley and Millie that they needed a new wire. He said that he and another lineman would put one in within the hour, and the electricity would be turned off during the installation. He turned and strode back down the hill to his truck. Within the hour the big truck came up the driveway, the electricity was turned off for a brief time, and a new wire was installed. Morley went out and asked why there had not been any problems with their electricity. The lineman told him it was because the insulation was frayed, not the wire itself, but they had been fortunate because, without insulation, problems would eventually occur.

After the men left, Morley and Millie shared their thoughts. They wondered why the lineman hadn't come to the door, rung the bell and told them what he found when he first walked up the driveway. Morley's truck and Millie's car were parked nearby, which might have suggested someone was home. The kitchen door with its lighted bell was only a few steps from the wire. The lineman had made no effort to talk with them. Had he done so, the situation would have been clarified because they would have shown him the frayed wire. It was only by chance that Millie had seen him. If she hadn't caught up with him he would have left. Had that happened, Millie would have telephoned the electric company again, restated that the wire was frayed, not repaired, and would have requested the lineman to return. They shook their heads over the added time that would have been involved. Oh well, at least a new wire now replaced the frayed one, the electricity had never shown a problem, and it was working fine now.

Morley half-chuckled, shook his head, turned to Millie and grumbled. "Millie, it's good you saw him and caught up to him, and I wouldn't have known it was only the insulation that was frayed, not the wire itself, if I hadn't asked him." He shook his head again. "So that's how they spend our tax money. They come to solve a problem, can't find one, plan to leave, don't give us information, or ask what we think."

* * *

It is not known what message the lineman received from the woman at the electric company. It is unclear whether she talked with him or just left a work order. Though she repeated to Millie that a frayed wire near the house was to be evaluated, the lineman didn't know he was supposed to evaluate a frayed wire. Even if he had not known because he had never received that information, or because he forgot, it was his responsibility to do a thorough check. Though we know he saw a short capped wire that he knew was no problem, but believed that was why Millie had called, he never considered talking with the McKerins to share his thoughts and ask for theirs. He returned to his truck, started writing his report, and planned to report back to the office. Orlando would have said he was behaving automatically from a belief that was not only an unrecognized assumption, but a belief that was an incorrect, unrecognized assumption.

When the lineman first evaluated the wire he could have come to the nearby door, rung the bell, told the McKerins what he found, and asked if the short capped wire was what had concerned them. Had he done this he would have been seeking verification as to whether or not his thoughts were correct. If he had talked with them that first time, which would have led him to reevaluate the wire, he would have revised his belief about the situation.

His automatic behavior did not include verifying the information he received. Deliberative behavior includes verifying before acting. Deliberative behavior also includes verifying your action to be sure the problem has been solved. He did not ask the McKerins if their electricity worked after he replaced the wire. It had not been a problem before, he was an expert in replacing wires, so it may not have occurred to him to check to be sure the electricity was working before he left.

Sometimes we behave from an unrecognized assumption that is correct. However, unless there is some form of verification, we don't know whether or not it is correct. Behavior carried out from incorrect assumptions can create problems. Obtaining verification can prevent problems.

Even though Orlando's Model includes five ingredients in successful communication, I believe validation (her term), translated here as verification, is the most important of the five ingredients.

The Model's ingredients flow one to another and can be remembered by their letters: PTFVA (Perceptions, Thoughts, Feelings, Validation, Action).

Perceptions are what we are aware of through our senses: what we see, hear, taste, touch, or smell. Another definition of perception includes an interpretation of what our senses are telling us, such as someone believing that a person is angry just by how he looks, rather than seeing that the person has a facial expression whose meaning is unclear. Orlando wants us to stay with the first definition. She believed it is important to be keenly aware of the perceptions we notice through our senses, because that is the first information we receive. The lineman's perception was accurate. He saw a short capped wire. Though someone else might add color, width, or something else specific about the wire, anyone looking at the wire would have agreed that it was a short capped wire.

Once we start interpreting what we have perceived, we are in the second and third ingredients: *Thoughts*, and/or *Feelings*. When the lineman saw the short capped wire he thought that was why the person had called. He knew it wasn't an electric wire, wasn't a problem, and whoever telephoned to have him evaluate a wire had made a mistake about this short capped wire being a problem. He had not thought beyond his interpretation, his belief that there was nothing more to check.

The story doesn't tell us what he may have felt when he thought the trip was unwarranted. We would be prudent not to assume any feelings he may have had. However, if we learned that he was annoyed about making a trip he considered unreasonable, we know those feelings would have been precipitated by thoughts that were inaccurate about the situation. We know the situation. He had made no effort to verify his inaccurate thoughts. He was writing his report and planning to leave.

Validation is the fourth ingredient. Verifying for accurate understanding of a situation is the only way we can know for sure whether or not we truly understand the situation. The lineman's verification about the situation occurred only because Millie ran after him and urged him to walk back up the driveway to reevaluate the wire she knew was frayed.

Action should only be taken after verification of the problem, and that action should be verified in order to ascertain whether or not it solved the problem. It appeared that the lineman was confident that replacing the frayed wire was an adequate solution, because he didn't return to ask the McKerins if the electricity was working after he turned it back on. However, we can never be sure an action solved the problem, or didn't cause another one, unless there is verification.

Orlando often told me she believed that it takes discipline to recognize one's assumptions, to verify one's thoughts and feelings for their reasonableness, and to verify the results of any action we may take. It did not occur to the lineman that he was making an assumption, that he had thoughts that needed verification. He believed it was reasonable to leave without getting any other information. If he had felt annoyed about thinking his trip to the McKerin Farm was unreasonable, those feelings would have come from his imagination about the situation, not from a situation whose accuracy he had verified. Until Millie clarified the situation and he reevaluated the wire, he was making and acting on an incorrect, inaccurate assumption.

Recognizing an assumption means that we are making a conscious effort to acknowledge that we are taking something for granted, accepting it as fact. To ascertain whether or not that assumption is true means making a further effort to obtain information that verifies. That is the only way to ensure that our thoughts, feelings, or actions are not arising from an incorrect interpretation of a situation. We are usually aware of our thoughts, but we are not always aware of our feelings. We can make the effort to recognize whether or not we are able to verify what we are thinking before and after taking an action, and whether or not any feelings are in response to our imaginations or in response to thoughts that have been verified for their accuracy. Thoughts we are unable to verify are only opinions. It is not reasonable to accept them as facts.

Orlando's Model is easy to understand, but can be deceptively difficult to do. Recognizing assumptions in complex and/or intense situations takes effort. Even though our first thoughts and feelings may occur almost immediately and may be fleeting, Orlando believed we need to capture them. When her students were working with patients, they would ask her what she would have done in a situation they described to her. Invariably her answer was the same. "This was your situation, not mine. You were there, I wasn't. What were your perceptions? What were you thinking? What were you feeling? How did you validate?" If needed, and if possible, she might send them back to the situation for more information. Frequently they struggled with remembering direct perceptions such as what was seen or heard. They also had difficulty remembering their first thoughts and feelings. It was more usual for them to describe their later thoughts and feelings with interpretations. I know this from having been one of her students. When I was a consultant to others who were trying to learn this process, the same struggle was evident.

Orlando emphasized that we needed to focus, be attentive, stay in the moment, not have our thoughts leap ahead. We'd sometimes work hard to remember what was occurring so we could relate the situation later when analyzing it with her. But when we did that, we'd forget more than we realized. She would remind us that if we stayed in the moment and were attentive to what was occurring, we would remember it. She gave a reasonable analogy. If someone stops us and tells a compelling story about a situation that takes our interest, we listen. We don't want to miss any of it. We may even make an attempt to be sure we have it right. "They really did that? Do I understand correctly that you mean . . . ?" If we're really interested we focus, stay attentive, and may even seek verification by our questions. When we do this we live in the situation. We become part of it. Then we usually remember it and get it right.

It is important, even crucial, to get it right when people's lives are at stake. People involved in programs that train doctors, nurses, and other health care professionals know this. They are aware that careful listening and effective communication that involves obtaining essential information needed for accurate diagnosis and treatment is not only basic to good patient care, it can also contribute to preventing medical errors.

Getting an accurate diagnosis means getting the story right. For treatment to be successful, it needs to be tailored to the individual patient. The following comment is from a neurologist. "No matter how many times I see the same disease, it seems to present itself not only differently, but uniquely, in each patient afflicted with it."[1] Even if the disease presentation seems remarkably similar and the treatment plan the same, how the patient accepts and follows that plan invariably has its own unique style and response. What patients think and feel affects their behavior. Communication skills of health care professionals can be crucial to successful outcomes.

Many books and articles on health care discuss the importance of the physician-patient relationship. Four of the most relevant books are: *Empathy and the Practice of Medicine*, by Howard Spiro, M.D., professor of medicine at the Yale University School of Medicine, and his colleagues; *Every Patient Tells a Story*, by Lisa Sanders, M.D., internist on the faculty of the Yale University School of Medicine; *How Doctors Think*, by Jerome Groopman, M.D., faculty in medicine at Harvard Medical School; and *Narrative Medicine*, by Rita Charon, M.D., Professor of Clinical Medicine, College of Physicians and Surgeons, Columbia University.[2]

Dr. Spiro writes: "doctors must listen to what the patient tells them, remaining open to be moved by the story even, for that will often clear the path to diagnosis. Listening goes straight to the heart and helps to create empathy . . . . The ear is as important as the eye in medical practice."[3] Dr. Sanders says that the patient's story is often the best place to find the clue that is needed in making a diagnosis. "It is our oldest diagnostic tool. And . . . it is one of the most reliable as well."[4] Dr. Groopman tells us his book is primarily written for laymen. "Because doctors desperately need patients and their families and friends to help them think. Without their help, physicians are denied key clues to what is really wrong."[5] Dr. Charon states: "A medicine practiced with narrative competence will more ably recognize patients and diseases, convey knowledge and regard, join humbly with colleagues, and accompany patients and their families through the ordeals of illness. These capacities will lead to more humane, more ethical, and perhaps more effective care."[6]

There are various programs for physicians in training which have at their core an emphasis on accurate observation and good communication skills. These programs include recognizing the importance of individualized patient care. However, some of those programs' administrators and faculty note various problems that need to be addressed. Though the following are only a few of those programs, they are examples of such training.

The first year medical students at the Yale University School of Medicine have classes on techniques of interviewing and doing physical exams from the beginning of that year. For the first two school years they meet weekly in small groups to review and practice these techniques. However, when Dr. Sanders attended a meeting with several directors from medical school and residency programs, one of the doctors stated a common complaint. Though students may do well when tested on their final exams at the end of their first and second years, their skills seem to be gone when they go into their clinical clerkships.[7]

One attendee told of a colleague who was pleased with a medical student's skills after having worked several times with him as his teacher. The student returned for one final class after some weeks into his first clerkship, a clerkship in internal medicine. This colleague observed the student evaluating a patient and was horrified to see him do everything wrong. He interrupted the patient's story. He asked closed-ended questions. He examined patients through their clothes, and he omitted much of the exam. This colleague could not believe the student's behavior was so different than what he had known of him. So he asked him what had happened. The student's answer was: "My resident says we don't have time to do all that. I mean, what's the point?"[8]

What's the point, indeed. Aren't our doctors supposed to take enough time to be thorough? If they are making diagnoses from incomplete physical exams and incomplete stories from their patients, is there not a greater chance of their acting on incorrect, unverified assumptions than if they are thorough and get the story right?

Dr. Irwin Braverman at the Yale School of Medicine, a professor of dermatology for over fifty years, had long been frustrated by his students' difficulty in describing their findings from examining skin. He was aware that astute observational skills are usually only acquired after several years of medical practice. He wanted to develop these skills much earlier. He knew the students learned patterns that represented different diagnoses, but they missed noticing what was odd, what was different than what they were used to seeing in the patterns. He realized they needed more training in careful, detailed observation. So he took them to Yale's Center for British Art in downtown New Haven, Connecticut, only a few blocks from the School of Medicine.

The medical students were encouraged to hone their powers of observation on paintings. They were to focus on each image in the paintings. Each painting had a story to tell. The students were to figure out what the story was and relate it to their classmates in concrete, descriptive terms. When they made interpretations from what they saw, they were asked how they derived those interpretations. "If you think a character looks sad, figure out what you are seeing that makes you think that and describe it. If you think that the picture suggests a certain place or class, describe the details that lead you to that conclusion." Results from testing the students' observational skills before and after spending an afternoon focusing on the paintings showed an improvement in their observations. As a result, the museum observations became a required class in the curriculum for Yale's first year medical students.[9]

The Yale School of Medicine is not alone in realizing that its students can improve on their observational skills from classes at art museums. Dr. Joel Katz's class of Harvard Medical School students meets at the Boston, Massachusetts, Museum of Fine Arts.[10] Medical classes at McMaster University, Hamilton, Ontario, Canada, view slides at the McMaster Museum of Art.[11] Professor Michael Baum, one of Britain's leading cancer experts, and a keen art critic, takes his medical students to the National Gallery in London, England.[12] Programs which include paintings to enhance medical students' observational skills appear to be increasing in many countries.[13]

Shimon M. Glick, M.D., at the Ben Gurion University Faculty of Health Sciences in Beer Sheva, Israel, states that communication skills are a major focus of their program for first year medical students. Their clinical sessions take place in various settings including a community clinic. Their discussions center almost exclusively on the patients' personal problems. Some students are hospitalized. In subsequent discussions with their classmates, they discuss and share their reactions to this experience. The students also meet with blind, deaf, and mentally retarded patients to learn about their problems including their struggles in interacting with others. Dr. Glick says the students are emotionally moved, and their empathy is significantly enhanced from their involvement with such patients.

In the second year the medical students have clinical weeks during which time they interview patients dying from cancer, patients who are surviving cancer, and family members. The goal is to have the students appreciate what it is like for patients and their families to experience such an illness. The students also spend a week with families in crisis by focusing on patients admitted to intensive care units. There they witness the impact of that situation on those patients and their families. Psychosocial aspects of medicine continue as a thread throughout the medical students' curriculum. Dr Glick states: "Dozens of anecdotal reports from patients, both hospitalized and in the community, have noted that Beer-Sheva graduates behave significantly more empathically than graduates of the other medical schools they have encountered."[14]

Jodi Halpern, M.D., Ph.D., who teaches ethics at the University of California Los Angeles (UCLA) Medical School, Los Angeles, California, believes physicians who have empathy are more successful with their patients than are those without empathy. She believes empathy helps physicians: understand how patients feel about their information while also timing their questions and tone in a way that invites communication; understand the subjective complaints of their patients; and understand the health values of their patients and their families in order to make a treatment plan that will be followed.[15]

In 1997 a hospital in Bangor, Maine, hosted the first book club for physicians, nurses, and other health care professionals to discuss medical themes in literature. By spring 2010 this idea had spread to twenty-five states including California, Florida, Massachusetts, Missouri, New York, Ohio, and Virginia. "The humanities can remind them that they're dealing with very complicated, whole individuals with their own needs and opinions," said Elizabeth Sinclair who is coordinator of the Maine Humanities Council's literature and medicine program. A 2005 study by the Maine Council showed that participants reported greater empathy for their patients and colleagues, more cultural awareness, increased job satisfaction, and improved interpersonal skills.[16]

Some programs other than those that train physicians have recognized the importance of including classes in observational skills, critical thinking, and consideration of what is involved in making a decision. The Yale University School of Nursing has classes at Yale's Center for British Art in New Haven for their graduate nursing students.[17] New York City police officers take a course titled The Art of Perception with Amy Herman, art historian and lawyer, at the Metropolitan Museum of Art. The course is designed to "fine tune their attention to visual details," and to consider how and why they make their decisions. Amy Herman's other students have included U.S. Secret Service agents, members of the Department of Homeland Security, the Transportation Security Administration, the Strategic Studies Group of the Naval War College, the National Guard, and, during a visit to London, the Metropolitan Police of Scotland Yard. Bill Reiner, FBI special agent, said: "Amy taught us that to be successful, you have to think outside the box. Don't just look at a picture and see a picture. See what is happening."[18]

The following are some of the business schools that have embraced critical thinking. The Graduate School of Business at Stanford University, Stanford, California, has a course for first year students titled Critical and Analytical Thinking. One of the issues their students entertain is: "In whose interest am I making the decision?" The Rotman School of Management at the University of Toronto, Toronto, Canada, has a course for first year students titled Fundamentals of Integrative Thinking. In their second year the course called The Opposable Mind focuses on developing and practicing the skills needed to be a good thinker and manager. One of the exercises involves practicing "assertive inquiry to explore the assumptions and validity of each executive's argument." An architectural firm in Seattle, Washington, finds the Rotman graduates free of the bias or predisposition that is often carried into situations. The Yale School of Management, New Haven, Connecticut, has a course to encourage their students to think more broadly, question assumptions, and "view problems through multiple lenses and learn from history."[19]

Training programs for professionals who are not aware of Orlando's Model, especially when they are involved with life and death matters, could improve upon their training by incorporating the Model into their programs. The Orlando Model takes discipline, but with effort, can be learned. The Model includes recognizing any assumptions made and ascertaining whether or not those assumptions are accurate. It requires staying in the moment, focusing attention, making detailed observations, capturing one's thoughts and feelings, and most of all, verifying whether or not there is an accurate understanding and accurate response to a situation. Thoughts we are unable to verify are not facts, they are opinions.

When others are involved, the Orlando Model requires awareness of whether or not one is on the same wave length with those others. In an effort to have clear and honest communication, empathy may also be necessary for others to feel they can offer honest information. Being on the same wave length enhances empathy.

The Orlando Model does not allow for automatic behavior. It requires us to think and behave with careful deliberation. The Model includes some of what the previous programs include, but those programs do not appear to include all the ingredients Orlando found relevant in successful communication and in adequately resolving situations: *Perceptions* that flow into *Thoughts* and/or *Feelings*, then *Validation* and *Action* with further *Validation*. Since the Orlando Model requires verification of one's thoughts, feelings, and actions, the Orlando Model incorporated into training programs for professionals in health care and elsewhere increases the probability of not only getting the story right, but also getting the action right.

20. Reflections

This chapter reflects on various issues inherent to, or prompted by, the stories. Innumerable stories reviewed for this book revealed a variety of issues. The stories chosen best portray those issues. Their contents led to the book's title and to the chapter titles. To fully appreciate the effect of assumptions, it is important to remember that an assumption is something we take for granted. We accept it as fact. As many of the stories show, we may or may not realize when we are making an assumption, let alone when we are acting on one. Since many stories include similar issues, it would be cumbersome to refer to all the stories that are relevant. Those left out are no less important than those that have been included.

Not long into the writing I began to realize that I am the messenger for the people in the stories. Whether in health care or elsewhere, the stories are about us. When we make, believe, and act on incorrect assumptions we can find ourselves in problematic, sometimes painful, situations. I am stunned at the degree to which we make and act out assumptions we don't even know we've made. The stories reveal that when our assumptions are incorrect, we can be led into situations that range from misunderstandings to deaths.

It appears that we are experts at premature closure. Too easily we can accept our immediate beliefs, expectations, or actions without any consideration of whether or not we are making assumptions that need to be verified. If it becomes apparent that these beliefs, expectations, or actions are based on incorrect assumptions, the resultant situations may take more time and involve more people before they are resolved, if they are ever resolved. They may be resolved, but not according to everyone's satisfaction. Where deaths are involved, it is too late.

In many of the stories incorrect assumptions occurred from quick decisive thinking followed by action with no thought of verifying whether or not the action made sense. It is striking that the people who were affected by those actions were right there, nearby, or could have been reached for their valuable information, if the effort had been made to hear what they had to say.

In the fire alarm story, the first story in the book, Mavis was a patient in the hospital unit where either Dr. McKay or the nurse who escorted her back to her room could have simply asked: "Mavis, why did you pull the alarm?" Either of them could have ascertained that she was no longer struggling with her admitting symptoms of confusion and hearing voices. She did not need to be transferred to a psychiatric hospital. She was doing what her mother had told her years ago: talk to a policeman or a fireman, or, if necessary, pull a fire alarm if you are lost and need help. She was merely trying to get help in finding out where she was that dark, predawn morning. But neither Dr. McKay nor the nurse asked her for her thoughts.

In the previous chapter, *Recognizing Assumptions*, Millie and Morley McKerin were in the house just a few feet from the wire the electric lineman evaluated. Like Dr. McKay and the nurse, it never occurred to him to include their thoughts. Had he believed it might be important to include them he would not have left so abruptly. He might have noticed vehicles near the house, noticed the nearby door, and rung the doorbell to see if anyone were there. Even if he thought they were mistaken about a small capped wire, he might have talked with them about what he found. They then could have informed him that they reported a frayed wire, not a small capped wire. This was another hasty decision without making any attempt to include the thoughts of those who were involved and available.

In Chapter 5, *Tenacious Assumptions, Dogged Beliefs*, there are two stories where those accused could have easily clarified the situation had there been an effort either to reach them or otherwise obtain the facts before making an incorrect assumption about them. These situations too often lead to misplaced gossip, and, if never corrected, such incorrect beliefs may be carried on for years. The first story is a classic he said-she said situation.

Harry planned to sue Jake, a mental health clinician and the clinic, because he believed Jake had said he was paranoid. Harry had heard this from Ada, Jake's patient, who told Harry that her therapist said he was paranoid. Zeke, Jake's administrator, did not read Jake's clinical note in Ada's chart, nor did he try to reach him because he was on vacation. Zeke told the Board that Jake and the clinic were being sued, as if it were a fact. Harry decided not to sue when he consulted a lawyer who told him that it was unlikely that any therapist would say that, and it was too soft a case. Even so, only after Jake returned, denied the accusation, and had Zeke read the chart did Zeke recant, albeit without an apology.

In the other story Alma was criticized for going to the movies by a woman who saw her entering the movie theater when her husband was a very ill patient in the local hospital. Alma had gone to see the newsreel because she had been told that their daughter, a medical intern, was in a medical scene in the news. Immediately after the newsreel she went to the hospital to share with her husband what she had seen. Alma never had any intent to stay for the movies. The next day she was told about this criticism by a close friend who dropped by for a visit. Alma clarified the situation with her friend, but it was never known whether the woman who had been critical ever knew that her criticism had not been based on fact.

If people offer information it may not be believed, it may not be considered important, or it may be understood differently than what the person means. When heard, however it is understood, it is not included as information that should be considered in clarifying, verifying, or reasonably resolving the situation.

In the inheritance story, also in *Tenacious Assumptions, Dogged Beliefs*, a lawyer's letter stated that, as heirs, Uncle Jacob's nephews should get together to sort out Uncle Jacob's real estate and personal property. Isaac vehemently kept accusing Aaron of wanting someone from the trust company to join them despite Aaron emphatically stating that those were not his thoughts, that he was only sharing the lawyer's letter for them to discuss, that he had no specific thoughts on the matter.

In a psychotherapy session I recall a young teenager telling me that her father believed she was on drugs which she had emphatically denied to him, as she did with me. But then she added, "I might as well go on drugs if that's what he thinks." He had pounced on her when he noticed that she slurred her speech some days when she came home from school. She had not been sleeping well, had not been eating an adequate lunch, or having a healthy snack mid-afternoon if she noticed her energy wane. When her sleep improved and she began to eat more reasonably, her slurred speech stopped, and her father stopped accusing her. Fortunately, despite the accusation, she did not go on drugs.

In the Virginia Tech shooting story in Chapter 4, *Urgent!*, the police ignored Heather's information that Emily and her boyfriend had an amazing relationship, that he was not violent, therefore he could not have shot Emily. Despite this information and without warning others on campus that a shooter might still be there, the police immediately left the campus to try to find him.

Also in *Urgent!*, Edna's cry of "I can't breathe!" was not considered important, relevant information. It was understood only in terms of what Keri, the conference leader, believed was reasonable behavior in reenacting a birth experience. This scenario is not all that different from the Dana Farber scenario in Chapter 1, *Orlando's Model*, where Betsy Lehman understood that she was in a critical situation without adequate response and, with the hope of getting some help, telephoned a friend who was a hospital social worker. It was too late for Edna and Betsy. They died.

Sometimes you are stopped from saying what you believe. You may be abruptly cut off before you have a chance to fully state your opinion and explain why your opinion is different. And so we find in Chapter 7, *Betrayed*, that first grade student Katie, age five-and-a half, is in tears telling her older brother that she flunked the test, but didn't understand why her answers were wrong. She told him she believed that a word that was "the same word" was not a reasonable answer to the question that asked what word was "the closest word" to the word on the other side of the page. As in all these above situations, it can be more than a minor frustration not to be believed when you know you are telling the truth. This situation for Katie was devastating. In tears she told her brother she feared flunking first grade.

Then there are situations where an action is carried out that affects you, but you have been given no opportunity to state your thoughts or feelings about it before it occurs. The assumption is made that your thoughts or feelings do not have to be considered. The assumption may not even be recognized. The story where Danny's mother gave her comic books to a summer fair when Danny was away at a summer camp was such a situation. It appeared that her mother never made any attempt to understand what the comic book trading activity meant to Danny, an activity so intimately involved with her friends. It appeared that she never considered that she might be doing something very hurtful. This story was also in Chapter 7, *Betrayed*.

Chapter 6, *Automatic Assumptions Can Mislead* includes a story about how easily stereotypical thinking can blind people to unique qualities of individuals. This was the situation when Susan Boyle came on the stage in "Britain's Got Talent" before she sang "I Dreamed a Dream" from *Les Miserables*. Stereotypical thinking is not usually so readily recognized, or so easily corrected.

Also in *Automatic Assumptions Can Mislead* are two stories where quick, incorrect, automatic assumptions led to tragic deaths. The first was the story about the man who was awakened at night by a noise in the bedroom. He saw an outline of a person, grabbed his gun, then shot and killed his fiancée. It was unclear whether or not he had told her there had recently been burglars in the neighborhood, and he planned to have his gun next to the bed. The other story was about the deer hunter who saw a white flash which he thought was the tail of a deer. He fired and instantly killed a woman who was in her yard hanging out her laundry. Actions triggered from quick, incorrect automatic assumptions, especially when one feels afraid, unsafe, and/or the adrenalin is flowing from an expectation or wish, can too easily lead to such tragedies.

When we automatically act on our beliefs or expectations without including all available information, it appears that it may not have occurred to us that our beliefs or expectations are unreasonable. As many of the stories have shown, if our assumptions are incorrect, we may find ourselves in regrettable situations that could have been avoided had we just taken the time to obtain more information.

Our beliefs and expectations come from our histories, also from the context in which we find ourselves. But when we leave out information from others who will be affected by our actions, whose agenda is it, theirs or ours? Whose needs, theirs or ours?

* * *

Mr. Kraus was admitted to the cardiac intensive care unit. Nurses were with him around the clock. The only time his wife left his side was when the nurses needed to attend to him. Even when the nurses made it clear that he was stabilized and in no danger, she continued to ignore the visiting hours. "I stay here," was her response to the suggestion that she leave and get some rest. As one nurse said to another: "She won't leave . . . . Eats a bit off his tray, won't even go downstairs to the cafeteria . . . . I've talked to her till I am blue in the face, but she won't go home. She just sits there in that straight wooden chair and holds his hand."

After two days one nurse finally said to her: "The heart attack was small . . . . He'll probably go home at the end of the week. You are exhausted . . . . You have not showered, not slept, nor have you eaten properly . . . . You'll be sick. You must go home to rest."

Mrs. Kraus listened politely. When the nurse stopped to take a breath Mrs. Kraus put her hand on the nurse's arm. With her other hand she pulled up her left sleeve showing a number tattooed on her arm. "The only time we were apart was at Auschwitz . . . . I would not have lived if he had not been there on the other side of the compound. When we were liberated, we made a promise never to leave each other again." She pulled down her sleeve then took her husband's hand. "I have not left him since, and I will not leave him now."

The nurse shared Mrs. Kraus' story with others at the nurses' station. Within minutes they took a basin and toiletries into the room so Mrs. Kraus could freshen up. A guest tray was ordered for supper. A sheet, pillow, and blanket were arranged in a lounger. In thirty minutes Mrs. Kraus was asleep next to her husband, their hands held tightly together. Later Mr. Kraus looked up at one of the nurses and in a soft voice said, "Thank you for finally listening." Then, while looking at his sleeping wife, he clearly, but still softly, added, "We have quite a story, Stella and I."[1]

* * *

In his book *Second Opinions*, Dr. Jerome Groopman described a nightmarish experience he and his wife, Dr. Pam Hartzband, had at the Children's Hospital, Boston, Massachusetts, where Steve, their nine-month-old child, was being evaluated for gastrointestinal symptoms.

It was a July 4th holiday weekend. They had flown from Los Angeles to New York, stayed the night at Pam's parents in Connecticut, and been dismissed by a pediatrician there who said

Steve's symptoms indicated an intestinal virus. As they left Pam's parents and drove toward Boston Steve fussed, would not drink any sugar water, and seemed worse. By dusk they reached their home not far from Boston. By mid-evening Steve's face was ashen. He was breathing in short gasps, desperately flexing his knees, and his arms were flailing. Pam yelled. "Let's take him to Children's Hospital—now!" After a frantic ride they arrived at Children's.

Despite a chaotic full waiting room, the triage nurse had them seen almost immediately. With flawless recall for detail, Pam described their son's relevant history and worsening symptoms to Dr. Scott Warren, their emergency room physician, a resident who was in his third postgraduate year of surgical training. However, by his questions it was obvious that Dr. Warren had not been carefully listening.

Then, suddenly, an intern, recognizable by his garb, came in with a grin, interrupted, and said, "What d'you got in here, Scott? What is it? A good case?" Dr. Groopman was livid and tore into him. "Who the hell are you? Who the hell are you? My son is not a 'good case'! My son is not an 'it'!" Dr. Groopman remembers he felt he might kill him. The intern looked at Dr. Groopman in shock, then, with a perplexed expression, looked at Dr. Warren. Dr. Groopman yelled at him. "Get out of the room! Now! Now!" Dr. Warren nodded to the intern to leave.

Steve's blood work indicated the possibility of major infection or tissue damage, and his X-rays confirmed the diagnosis of intussusception of the bowel, a very grave situation. "I guess you're going to operate to relieve the obstruction," Pam said as she looked at Dr. Warren. "In my clinical experience we can safely observe your son overnight. It's premature to operate. And it's already past midnight," was his reply. Then he told them that since they were physicians they were welcome to the coffee by the nurses' station, that he was leaving to see a couple more kids, and he hoped to get some sleep. Dr. Groopman glanced at the clock. It was12:17 a.m.

"I don't trust him," said Pam. Their son was deteriorating. His skin was mottled. He was hotter to their touch. His eyes were glazed, and hardly moving. Dr. Groopman felt a sense of dread. Both agreed that it didn't feel safe to wait. Dr. Groopman struggled to think of someone to call. Then he remembered having had some basic science training in Dr. David Nathan's department. Physicians' home phones are not always listed. Fortunately Dr. Nathan's was, so Dr. Groopman got the number from the operator and telephoned from the bustling emergency room pay phone. Apologizing for the late call, Dr. Groopman described the situation and asked for help. Dr. Nathan said he'd call Dr. Ray Levy, and Dr. Levy would contact Dr. Warren. Dr. Groopman recognized the name. Dr. Ray Levy was one of the most renowned pediatric surgeons in the country.

No more than ten minutes later Dr. Warren came into the examination room and flatly informed Dr. Groopman that Dr. Levy was driving in from his home. Not long thereafter Dr. Levy, a tall, portly, slightly gray haired man with delicate hands, arrived and greeted the parents with no hint of annoyance at being called in the middle of the night and on a holiday weekend. He obtained the needed history from Pam, examined Steve, and intently studied the X-rays. He explained to the worried parents that their son needed emergency surgery. If Steve's bowel burst he might die. Waiting until morning increased that risk. Both parents signed a consent form they barely read.

Walking with the nurse, Dr. Levy guided the stretcher to the operating room. After the operation Dr. Levy explained that "the bowel was ashen, moments from perforating." The operation was just in time, no resection was necessary, and nothing else was found. Dr. Levy told them Steve would be in the intensive care unit on antibiotics and should be home by the end of the week, also that he'd see him midday. With tears Dr. Groopman and his wife thanked Dr. Levy who clasped Dr. Groopman's hand and seemed almost embarrassed by the gratitude.[2]

* * *

So indeed, whose agenda, whose needs are being met? Especially if we feel strongly about a situation, what does it take for us to be heard?

Mrs. Kraus stayed firm and would only leave her husband's side when the nurses were attending to him. They kept pressing her to go home and get some rest. "I stay here," was her firm reply. When she finally told one nurse about being in Auschwitz, that she and her husband had promised never to leave each other again, the nurses no longer pressed her to leave and did what they could to make her stay more pleasant. Though Mr. Kraus thanked the nurse "for finally listening," the nurses would not have understood if Mrs. Kraus had not told one of them why she would not leave. Dr. Groopman and his wife knew that their emergency room physician was not carefully listening to the detailed description about the progressively deteriorating condition of their nine-month-old son. Even when the blood tests supported the possibility of a serious condition, and the X-rays confirmed the grave diagnosis of intussusception of the bowel, Dr. Warren still didn't consider the situation an emergency.

When Dr. Groopman told their lay friends about this experience, they said, "What if you and Pam weren't doctors?" He acknowledged the point, but he wants us to know that they didn't think about using a professional connection until they stopped being passive. He emphasized that it's important to speak up if we sense that something is seriously wrong with someone we know so intimately. Regarding Dr. Warren, he added: "We doubted his competence because we saw that he was not focused on Steve, that he was tired, distracted, and eager to sleep, and that his decision was couched in the arrogance of limited experience."[3]

Knowing someone intimately may be knowing a family member, a close friend, or knowing yourself and your symptoms when the situation involves you. In Chapter 14, *When We Are Patients* are three such stories.

In the first story I sensed I was being dismissed at Yale University Health when the physician couldn't find anything in my eye that made it feel scratchy. I made it clear I would not leave with the problem unresolved. Although he was stern and seemed reluctant, he sent me upstairs to an ophthalmologist who pulled out a very tiny, almost invisible eyelash that had gone under my eyelid. In the second story Pamela Gallin, M.D., a surgeon, needed surgery on her right hand, her operating hand, so she chose the best surgeon possible. Post operatively she was in severe pain from her hand which had been put in a cast. She telephoned her surgeon who reassured her that she was fine and promised that the pain would go away. With her pain worsening and her fingers swelling, she knew she was not fine. Even though she telephoned her surgeon's office for the next three days and stated her situation, she was not given an appointment.

A radiologist friend told her to demand to be seen. So when she telephoned her surgeon's office to be seen and was told he was out of town, she said she'd see someone else. The surgeon who removed her too tight cast appeared furious when he first saw her swollen hand, then found an incision that had popped open and swelling that had impeded the blood supply and crushed some nerves. It took six months for the nerves to regrow. For the next two years she underwent two scar revision surgeries. Each time her hand was in a cast for a month. None of this would have been necessary had her surgeon listened, treated her with respect, and seen her when she first told him she had a lot of pain.

She admitted that her surgeon's lack of response made her feel like a bad patient. In retrospect she thought that if she, a surgeon, were too intimidated to confront her doctor when she sensed something wrong, then it must be more difficult for people not involved in health care to speak up when someone in authority is questioning them. If we are in a situation that involves our health and we think something is wrong, she encourages us to refuse to take no for an answer when we wish to be seen.

In the third story Ellen O'Connor refused to accept the recommendation of exploratory surgery for Sandra, her daughter, from an intern when she was aware that her daughter's condition was improving. Ellen said her daughter felt less feverish, was no longer cranky, and she had become more like her usual self. When the intern thought X-rays of Sandra's abdomen indicated possible intussusception of the bowel, Ellen asked him if he thought or knew this. He did not respond with a straight answer. She felt he was not listening when he kept insisting that Sandra be taken for surgery. When she asked what other tests could prove his suspicion of intussusception he said ultrasound, but it would require a specialist to come in to do the test. Neither she nor her husband relented. The specialist who gave them a hard time when he came in to do the ultrasound was as surprised as the intern that the ultrasound showed that Sandra's intestines were moving normally. Sandra had viral gastroenteritis, an infection, not intussusception of the bowel.

Ellen admitted it was a hard decision for her and her husband to question the doctors. But she felt that she knew her child and, since Sandra's symptoms had improved, both she and her husband believed they should not accept exploratory surgery when they found that a less invasive informative test was available. We, too, should ask if there are less invasive informative tests available if we are offered exploratory surgery as a way to confirm a diagnosis.

The Orlando Model requires health professionals to take seriously what patients or their surrogates say. As responsible, concerned parents who knew their children well, Dr. Groopman and his wife and Ellen O'Connor and her husband were able to state clear information about the changing symptoms of their very seriously ill children. Those parents knew that the physicians responsible for evaluating and making decisions about their children were not carefully listening.

Dr. Gallin, as a patient, was well able to state her symptoms, as was I. Neither of us were seen by physicians who could solve our problems until we refused to be dismissed. Neither of our assigned physicians believed what we had to say.

As previously stated in Chapter 12, *Our Doctors Need Our Stories*, Lisa Sanders, M.D. noted in her book, *Every Patient Tells a Story*, that the patient's story is not only the oldest diagnostic tool, it is often the best place to find the clue that unravels the mystery. Also referenced in that chapter, Sir William Osler, M.D., the father of modern medicine, told his medical students that "the best teaching is that taught by the patient himself." Dr. Groopman believes that patients can offer the most vital information about themselves which can steer their physicians toward the correct diagnosis and relevant therapy, thereby helping even the most seasoned physicians to avoid errors in thinking.[4]

The Institute of Medicine Report, *To Err Is Human*, the report focusing on patient safety and avoiding errors, states that "patients should be a part of the care process" which includes "their own knowledge of their condition."[5] Yet here we have three physicians, Dr. Groopman and Dr. Hartzband, as patient surrogates reporting on the continuing deterioration of their son, and Dr. Pamela Gallin, as a patient reporting on her deteriorating condition, and even their information is dismissed.

As also noted in Chapter 12, both Dr. Sanders and Dr. Groopman believe that the most common diagnostic errors involve how doctors think. Both are concerned with physicians' failing to question their assumptions, ignoring data that doesn't fit, and shortcut thinking through pattern recognition, algorithms, stereotypes, and biases, any of which can lead to premature closure.[6]

It is striking how often premature closure from incorrect assumptions in both health care and elsewhere is preventing us from getting the story right. It seems incredible how often those stories where incorrect assumptions were made and incorrect actions carried out involved participants whose invaluable information, though easily available, was not sought, or if obtained was either not believed, was denied, ignored, or just misunderstood.

One of the reasons for premature closure can be an intolerance for uncertainty. Jay Katz in *The Silent World of Doctor and Patient* believes that there is "the universal human tendency to turn away from uncertainty" and, for physicians, training for certainty begins in medical schools.[7] Though beliefs and expectations without verification can result in incorrect assumptions, this universal tendency to avoid uncertainty may account for some of the premature closures that not only occur in health care, but also elsewhere. Avoiding uncertainty can create unexpected results.

* * *

A hospital intern needed to make a decision about the dose of a medication. He recognized the patient's condition and which medication to use. But the medication was used in different dosages for a number of conditions, and he didn't know the correct dose for this patient's condition. Should he interrupt his supervising resident during a meeting to ask about the dose, or should he guess? He guessed. This could have resulted in adverse effects. Fortunately there were none.[8]

* * *

An intern in medical training was surprised that she had received a low grade from her supervising physician. She knew she was one of the best interns in her group, so she asked for an explanation. He told her his reason was that she didn't know as much as the others. From her experiences with her peers she knew she was one of the most knowledgeable, not the least. So she asked him what evidence had led him to that conclusion. His reply: "You ask more questions."[9]

* * *

A Hollywood talk show producer told a story about flying with her father in his private airplane which was running out of gas and he was uncertain about the location of the landing strip. She began to panic and said, "Daddy! Why don't you radio the control tower and ask them where to land?" His response: "I don't want them to think I am lost."[10]

* * *

On Friday, June 17, 1994, a computer problem prevented Fidelity Investments from calculating the value of 166 mutual funds. Instead of reporting that the values for these funds were not available, a manager reported to the National Association of Securities Dealers that the values of these funds had not changed from the previous day. However, because June 17 was a down day in the financial markets, the values of Fidelity's funds that were published were noticeably higher than other published funds. This resulted in a cost and inconvenience to brokerage firms because they had to recompute their customers' accounts. This false reporting was also an injustice to investors who made buy or sell decisions based on inaccurate information. In an attempt to put some closure on this embarrassing situation, Fidelity was forced to make a public apology.[11]

* * *

These stories show only some of the various ways people avoid uncertainty. The hospital intern dealt with uncertainty by guessing. The woman medical intern asked questions. Whether or not her peers knew more because they did not ask as many questions is unclear. Maybe one of the reasons they received higher grades was because they did not put themselves in the position of appearing uncertain. The pilot refused to call the radio tower because he didn't want anyone there to know he was uncertain about the landing strip's location. The financial manager lied instead of being honest and admitting that the funds' values were not available because of a computer problem. That was his way of not appearing to be uncertain.

Not admitting uncertainty can result in a wide range of consequences in health care and elsewhere. As noted in Chapter 16, *Hospitals and Hierarchies*, the airlines realized they had to support their flight crews for speaking up when they are uncertain or if they are aware something is amiss. Such information can be essential in recognizing and solving problems, some of which could otherwise lead to disastrous airline accidents with loss of life.

As also noted in Chapter 16, patient safety is improved when hospitals level their hierarchies, as have the airlines, by considering all staff at all levels as important members whose information is valuable in recognizing and solving problems. As noted in that chapter, Dr. Pronovost and his team leveled the usual hierarchy by including executives in unit teams so they would better understand and contribute to recognizing and solving problems. Problems were revealed and solutions found when the unit staff realized that these teams were sincere in wanting honest communication.

* * *

In March 2005 in a veterans hospital in Pittsburgh, Pennsylvania, surgeon Dr. Jon Lloyd, industrial engineer Peter Perreiah, and Tufts University nutritionist Jerry Sternin and his wife, Monique, joined together as leaders with a plan to lower infections of methicillin-resistant staphylococcus aureus (MRSA), a very serious infection that can cause deaths. Despite attempts to lower the rate of these infections, there had been years without adequate progress. They knew that the Sternins had been successful in reducing malnutrition in children in Vietnam only after they included the villagers in solving the problem. They wanted to follow a similar plan.

They held a series of thirty minute small group discussions with health care workers at every level: food service workers, janitors, nurses, doctors, and patients. They said: "We're here because of the hospital infection problem, and we want to know what *you* know about how to solve it." Ideas poured out. Many of them said it was the first time anyone had ever asked them what to do. When new hand-gel dispensers arrived, the staff put them up where they believed they should go. Nurses began to tell the doctors to wash their hands if they failed to do so. Other ideas, including wearing gloves in certain circumstances, were instituted. Nasal cultures were taken from every hospital patient upon admission and upon discharge. Their ideas and progress were published on the hospital Web site and in newsletters. The monthly results, unit by unit, were posted. One year into the experiment the entire hospital's MRSA wound infection rates dropped to zero.[12]

* * *

Chapter 16 also noted that Dr. Pronovost and Dr. Gawande have shown that relevant, concise checklists used with good judgment lower rates of infection and thereby improve patient safety. However, for checklists to work, the staff need to own them, be part of them, contribute to them, and refine them as needed. Chapter 17, *Hierarchies*, included Dr. Gawande's visit to a construction site where he learned about the construction industry's methods of ensuring safety when they build major hospital buildings and large, complicated high rise structures. They assume anything can go wrong. The hierarchy includes various levels of authority and expertise. Everyone along the way is responsible for ensuring safety. Checklists make sure that simple steps are not missed. They have another set of checklists to make sure that everyone talks through and resolves any conceivable, or unexpected problems. Like the airline industry, they know one minor problem can have an untoward domino effect.

Leaders need to realize that their behavior has a huge effect in establishing the emotional tone of an organization. When Pam Brier became a hospital administrator at Jacobi Medical Center, a public hospital in the Bronx, New York, she first walked around Jacobi and shook hands with every person who was there. Then she took almost every single doctor out to lunch or dinner and, with paper and pencil, took notes.[13] When Susan Hockfield became president of the Massachusetts Institute of Technology, Cambridge, Massachusetts, one of the first things she did was go on a listening tour.[14] Drew Gilpin Faust, President of Harvard University, said, "An enormous amount of my job is listening to people, to understand where they are, how they see the world so that I can understand how to mobilize their understanding of themselves in service of the institutional priorities."[15]

People feel valued and offer more creative thinking and effective solutions when they work in a culture that encourages good listening and free flowing communication at all levels. We saw this in Chapter 17, *Hierarchies*, at Gore Associates which functions without a hierarchy. We saw this in Chapter 18, *The Milieu in Health Care*, at Hospice, which has the patients' needs as its core focus.

As there is a human need to avoid uncertainty, there is a human need to feel in control, and to feel that what will occur is predictable. Those in a position to take charge and make decisions should realize that this is no less so for people who have major physical, mental, or emotional struggles. They not only deserve to be heard, they may be able to contribute to our understanding of their situations, and sometimes they offer relevant solutions.

* * *

Though Brunhilde was her name, and most people called her Hilde, she knew that many people called her "the crazy one." She had psychotic symptoms which sometimes showed when she mumbled unintelligible thoughts or when she admitted hearing voices no one else heard. She knew the voices were only in her head, but she wouldn't tell her psychiatrist because she feared he'd put her back in the hospital.

Now she had come to visit her son-in-law and her pregnant daughter who would probably be delivering within a couple weeks. Arguments between her and her son-in-law escalated during the first few days. The police were summoned because, said another family member, she had begun to talk "crazy," and she had hit her son-in-law. The police called in mental health.

The person from mental health listened, making sure to hear Brunhilde's version of the situation. "So," asked the mental health clinician, "what do you think is the problem?" She admitted that she and her son-in-law had never gotten along. She added that she couldn't handle being around her daughter with the impending birth. "What do you think is the solution?" he asked. "It'd probably be better if I went home." He nodded. "How are you going to get there?" She said she could take the bus, but she didn't have enough money. Her son-in-law offered to pay, and take her to the bus. That was fine with her. Brunhilde had come by bus, knew the route, and she admitted she would prefer to be home with Muffins, her cat a friend had been taking care of while she was away. Her daughter went with them to the bus stop. The good-byes were pleasant and peaceful. Brunhilde hugged her daughter who promised to stay in touch by phone.

* * *

A thirty-eight-year-old patient in a psychiatric hospital with a history of more than twenty years of violent episodes was in such a rage that the other patients were evacuated from the room. The plan was to forcibly medicate her, but the male nurse requested talking with her before using force. As he opened the door she raised her head and looked almost like a wild beast about to attack an intruder. He went to her, acknowledged her by saying her first name, then softly, and with sympathy, told her he realized she was going through one of her bad moments, that she had to be medicated, but he didn't want to see her forcibly held down. She remained silent. Then she asked him if he would do it. He said he would. A couple male nurses' aides stood by as he gave her the injection. About forty-five minutes later she came and apologized to him for her unbecoming behavior.[16]

* * *

You may remember Alicia whom I buddied in a psychiatric unit when she was running around the room in an acute manic psychotic episode. She was in the first story in Chapter 10, *Acknowledge Me.* She, too, once she gained control, later apologized for her out-of-control behavior. Though I had offered her ginger ale and otherwise tried to communicate with her, I thought I had failed to reach her until later when she apologized for her "nasty" behavior. She well remembered being with me. "You were the only buddy who offered me anything. You were the only buddy who got me some ginger ale," she poignantly reminded me.

Chapter 10 included stories of others who were aware of reality, though that awareness was not at first validated by them. When Dillon and Whitley, in the acute care unit of a psychiatric hospital, were struggling with confused thinking, Mrs. MacGregor told them her name, and that the medication she was giving them would help them think better. When their thinking became clear they told her they remembered what she had said. Sam, the eighty-eight-year-old geriatric hospital patient with progressive dementia, calmed down and joined in his care when the staff realized that they needed to go where he was, namely to his shoe shop. When they gave him some old shoes to work on, he joined in with his care and did his own range-of-motion exercises. Sarah, the five-year-old child with autism, joined in with her care when the physician's assistant focused on her, not on her mother, explained what he was going to do, and had her assist him in her examination.

As noted in Chapter 18, *The Milieu in Health Care*, some of the sixty-five to ninety-year-old residents of Arden House, a nursing home, were given more control over their lives when they individually chose a plant to take care of and chose which of two nights they preferred to watch the movie. They were reminded about the many ways they could choose to spend their time, such as visiting with other residents, reading, listening to the radio, or watching television. When compared to the group not given those choices, these residents interacted more with other residents and staff, over 90% had improved physical health, and six months later were less likely to have died.

We do better when we are supported in taking charge of our lives. Remember Carmella in Chapter 9, *The Need to be Heard*, who, in her early psychotherapy sessions kept deferring to what her mother said or thought when I asked for her thoughts? She had entered therapy with a depression that included prolonged slowness when removing or putting on her coat, hat, and mittens, and she responded to my questions with "my mother says," or "my mother thinks." With encouragement and support, slowly, over time, when she became more comfortable thinking on her own and sharing her thoughts, her depression lifted, and she planned to join a reading group at the library.

Also in Chapter 9 were Maria and Tammy with their mothers in the toy store, and little Willie who began to talk nonstop when he was around three. Maria's mother supported Maria's wish to get a doll that does various things, such as one that wets, cries, and laughs. Tammy's mother told her she could have a better doll, a doll that listens. It was Tammy who was talking to her doll as she walked through the cashier's aisle and on toward the escalator, not Maria, who was focused on how to make her doll do what it was designed to do, but needed water for the doll and some assistance from her mother when they got home.

In order to develop a unique and stable identity children need others to understand and appreciate what they uniquely think and feel. Adults who think for and do for their children when their children only need encouragement and support to learn for themselves, deprive their children of their need to learn how to think through and handle situations on their own. As soon as we are able, we need to hear ourselves think to know more clearly what we think and feel and to sort it all out. This includes handling different situations with the support of caring adults, not having the adults do it for us.

The stories about the little children in Chapter 7, *Betrayed*, are especially poignant when we remember that those children found themselves in unexpected situations which left them in tears. Little five-and-a-half-year-old Katie was reprimanded because she didn't answer the test about the closest word according to what Miss Bristle believed was correct. Ten-year-old Danny came home from summer camp and abruptly learned that her mother had given her comic books to a fair. Someone left two-year-old Gina alone with her little suitcase in the hospital cafeteria. Do we really believe the thoughts and feelings of little children shouldn't be better considered in situations that involve them? Should we really leave them out and believe we got the story right?

Little Sarton, named after the author May Sarton, had a good relationship with May. She and May were in May's car one day when Sarton said, "It is very hard to be five. So much is expected of you."[17] Children, sometimes even more than adults, have a need to be heard and understood, and need some certainty, control, and predictability in their lives. The atmosphere of a milieu is affected by the people who are there, but no more so than by those on whom we depend.

Premature closure can occur if we think within the box, think narrowly from our beliefs and expectations without including all possible, relevant information. This type of thinking occurred in many of the stories where incorrect assumptions were made and actions were inappropriately carried out. Our beliefs and expectations may be correct for a situation. However, without verification we don't know whether or not our thoughts or actions are reasonable. Some situations cannot be resolved by conventional thinking.

* * *

On August 5, 1949, one of the hottest days ever recorded in Montana, a fire was reported at Mann Gulch. Mann Gulch is part of a geological transition where the Great Plains meet the Rocky Mountains. The gulch runs into the lower end of a spectacular stretch of the Missouri River. That summer the grass was especially tall, the timber very dry. The fire, caused by lightning, began in a heavily timbered area near the top of a ridge. Fifteen Smokejumpers parachuted in from a small plane with Wag Dodge as the crew foreman.

Dodge moved his Smokejumpers along the side of the gulch. A breeze was blowing the flames away from them. Suddenly the wind reversed. Dodge saw the fire leapfrog across the gulch and spark the grass below them. An updraft began. Fierce winds howled through the canyon as the fire sucked in the surrounding air. In seconds the fire began to devour the grass. The new fire coming up the gulch toward the men was coming faster than they were going.

The men started running up the slope toward the ridge. Dodge lit a match and ignited the grass on the uphill side of him. The flames were quickly moving up the slope. Dodge yelled to the men running by to join him. They did not. He stepped into his fire surrounding himself by a buffer of burned land. He wet his handkerchief with his canteen water, covered his mouth with the cloth, then lay down on the smouldering embers. He closed his eyes and inhaled the thin layer of oxygen clinging to the ground. He waited for the main fire to pass over him. Dodge survived. Two of the Smokejumpers found openings and reached the top of the ridge. They survived. The other Smokejumpers didn't make it. Their bodies lay scattered over the gulch. Later, Dodge was asked if he had "ever been instructed in setting an escape fire," Dodge replied, "Not that I know of. It just seemed the logical thing to do."[18]

* * *

The physician's assistant (P.A.) was working the night shift when the paramedics rushed in with a young man whose arm was severely bleeding from deep lacerations. An artery had been cut, which was believed to have happened when the patient had punched his arm through a glass shower door during an argument with his girlfriend. The patient reeked of alcohol and was yelling profanities. As the P.A. began to suture, the patient cursed again. "Damn it! That hurts. What the hell are you doing?" The P.A. calmly explained that he was suturing the wound so he wouldn't bleed to death. "Ow! It feels like my arm was just zapped—like you did something to my funny bone!" The P.A. quickly responded, "Don't worry. You'll be fine. This is normal." He finished treating the wound and left the room, hoping never to see this patient again.

Three days later the patient returned complaining of numbness and pain in his fourth and fifth fingers. "What did you do to me? Something is wrong with my hand." The P.A. examined the wound and told him that the discomfort was a normal part of the healing process. After the pain and numbness deteriorated into paralysis of his fourth and fifth fingers, the patient consulted a hand surgeon. The surgeon said there was significant damage to the ulnar nerve and recommended exploratory surgery. That surgery revealed that a suture used to tie off the bleeding vessels tied off the ulnar nerve which was then deprived of oxygen and blood flow, causing the nerve to die. A second surgery was needed to repair the problem.

The patient sued. His lawyer contacted the hand surgeon and asked, "If my client's nerve damage had been recognized when he first returned to the hospital complaining of numbness, would this injury have been reversible?" "Absolutely," said the surgeon. "It would have been much easier to treat closer to the time it happened. Basically, his ulnar nerve was dying right before the eyes of the hospital staff." The P.A. realized that the patient's complaint about feeling like someone had "zapped" his funny bone and the subsequent numbness of his fourth and fifth fingers should have been a clue to the problem. The case was settled out of court for $275,000.[19]

* * *

Conventional thinking that comes from one's beliefs and expectations can too easily narrow the focus and result in thoughts and actions that have not included information that is different, information that is not expected. The unusual information is ignored and the familiar solution that worked before is chosen. Maybe we are more likely to go on automatic when we are in intense, emergency situations that call for decisive, immediate action. But maybe that is just when we need to be more vigilant, more alert, more conscious of all available information. In both these stories the unexpected information that was there was ignored because it didn't fit in with what was believed: the men running by Dodge and his escape fire didn't understand what Dodge was doing; the P.A. ignored the patient's complaint that the P.A. had done something to his funny bone. Even when the patient returned and said that something was wrong with his hand, a situation that no longer seemed urgent, the P.A. denied the importance of the comment. This is similar to Pamella Galen, M.D., in Chapter 14, *When We Are Patients*, trying to get her surgeon to respond to her post surgical symptoms of unrelenting, severe pain in her hand that was in a cast.

We are more comfortable when we feel certain and find life predictable. We don't like to make mistakes. If we make them, we find it difficult to own up to them.

* * *

Twenty executives at a conference for the National Council of Nonprofit Associations were in a seminar titled Mistakes. They were to tell a mistake they had made as a leader. They were not to say how they had corrected it or avoided responsibility for it. Despite those rules, participants became uncomfortable and would try to tell a redeeming anecdote about a success or recovery from the mistake. By about the halfway point these executives were admitting major errors, such as failing to get a grant request in on time which cost the organization hundreds of thousands of dollars in lost revenue. About a half hour into the session laughter became so loud and raucous, "that nearly hysterical laughter of release of a great burden," that attendees from other seminars came into this seminar to see what the commotion was all about.[20]

* * *

In November 1999, Linda Kenney, age thirty-seven, was admitted to Brigham and Women's Hospital, Boston, Massachusetts, for ankle replacement surgery. Linda, born with club feet, believed that her surgery would be uneventful. Instead, a nerve block injected by Dr. Rick van Pelt, anesthesiologist, went straight to her heart, sending her into full-blown cardiac arrest. She was saved by open heart surgery. When she regained consciousness in the intensive care unit (ICU) she wanted to know what went wrong. A nurse told her that she probably had an allergic reaction to the anesthesia. She didn't believe it.

It is not certain what exactly happened, but Dr. van Pelt believes that the most likely explanation is that the needle inadvertently punctured a vein. He had not been clumsy or inattentive. He did not believe he made an error. However, he said, "I was responsible, I had created a horrible adverse event with a standard procedure."

Linda was not offered an explanation and felt abandoned by the hospital. Dr. van Pelt could not suppress the trauma he felt, so he sent her a letter of apology in which he offered to talk. Six months later they met. He told her what happened. She also believed that he did not make an error. She offered her doctor forgiveness. "That was a very profound moment. I felt like I had my life back," he said.

After that they teamed up to speak about their experience and to open lines of communication for those involved in such incidents. In 2002, Linda launched Medically Induced Trauma Support Services, a nonprofit service that provides support to anyone involved in an adverse event. Dr. van Pelt talked to Brigham administrators about the need to acknowledge the impact errors can have on patients and staff. The hospital launched the Peer Support Team Initiative, which connects doctors and nurses with their colleagues after adverse events and offers them a safe environment where they can discuss what happened and receive emotional support. Brigham became a leader in patient safety and in openness when things go wrong.[21]

* * *

As noted in Chapter 16, *Hospitals and Hierarchies*, the Institute of Medicine Report, *To Err is Human*, estimated that between 44,000 and 98,000 patients died from medical errors in

U.S. hospitals in 1997. These numbers were extrapolated from some studies in hospitals in Colorado, Utah, and New York. In those studies the Report noted that over half of the adverse events resulted from medical errors that could have been prevented.[22]

Dr. Atul Gawande states that 98% of American families that are hurt by medical errors don't sue.[23] Analyses of malpractice lawsuits have shown that there are highly skilled doctors who are sued a great deal and doctors who make many mistakes who are never sued. Patients sue when they feel they have been rushed by their doctors, or when they feel that their doctors have ignored them or treated them poorly. As Alice Burkin, a leading medical malpractice lawyer, said, "People just don't sue doctors they like."[24]

Wendy Levinson, a medical researcher recorded hundreds of conversations between a group of physicians and their patients. About half of the doctors had never been sued. The surgeons who had never been sued were more likely to make comments about what would happen, such as, "First I'll examine you, and then we will talk the problem over." They were also more likely to show active listening such as, "Go on, tell me more about that." Those surgeons spent on average three minutes longer with their patients. There was no difference in the amount or quality of information they gave. The recorded conversations were judged according to qualities such as warmth, hostility, dominance, and anxiousness. If the surgeon's voice sounded dominant, the surgeon tended to be in the sued group. If the surgeon's voice sounded less dominant and more concerned, the surgeon tended to be in the non-sued group. The difference was in how they talked with their patients. In effect, those who were not sued actively listened and showed respect by not talking down to their patients.[25]

A British report on malpractice noted that an original injury is not enough to cause a malpractice suit. Insensitive handling and poor communication are also required. More than a third of the group studied would not have litigated if they had received an explanation or apology.[26] Studies of hospitals in the United States have found that patients are less likely to sue when doctors admit and apologize for their mistakes and when changes are implemented so future patients will not be similarly harmed. "Being assured that it won't happen again is very important to patients," says Lucien Leape, a physician and professor of health policy at the Harvard School of Public Health."[27]

Our physicians may not realize that their relationship with us is very important to us. We are dependent on them for their knowledge and skill, also for believing that they care. So if they make a mistake, it is not so surprising that we prefer an explanation and an apology rather than being left with the feeling that we have been abandoned when they offer no information.

Chapter 13, *How We Hear Our Doctors*, includes stories that show the dramatic effect our physicians' words can have when we are severely ill. Mr. Wright's cancer remitted only as long as he believed that his physician believed that the Krebiozen injections would offer a cure. The woman who had improved and was doing well a year after receiving laetrile treatment for a malignant brain tumor died the same night after she unexpectedly came upon her original physician who expressed shock and surprise about her treatment, and declared it to be worthless. Two patients misunderstood the meaning of the cardiac terms their physicians used. TS meant tricuspid stenosis, not a life threatening situation, but that patient thought it meant terminal situation. She died. A wholesome gallop was a bad sign, a sound caused by a failing left ventricle straining ineffectively to pump blood, but that patient misunderstood wholesome gallop to mean a healthy gallop. He thought he was not dying, and he dramatically improved.

The last two stories in that chapter were endearing as much because of the warm relationship between the patients and their doctors as for the outcomes. Tony lived twelve years beyond the diagnosis of end stage cardiomyopathy by positively responding to his doctor's two five-year contracts. It is true that Tony wanted to live longer, but it is also important that the contracts worked because Tony believed and trusted in his doctor's expertise. Dr. Kronberg gave Joe, the renowned director of Canterbury's rare book library, a reason to live when he prescribed "One set of memoirs."

As also noted in Chapter 13, the mind's influence on our physical health is well documented in the research from psychoneuroimmunology (PNI). Hope and positive belief can promote healing. Lack of hope and feelings of helplessness can lead to death. We should never assume that our minds do not have an effect on our health and our ability to function. In this regard is a story about Pablo Casals, the famous cellist.

* * *

Norman Cousins met Pablo Casals for the first time at his home in Puerto Rico a few weeks before his ninetieth birthday. Because Pablo struggled with various infirmities, it was difficult for him to dress himself, so his wife helped him start his day. As he came into the living room on the arm of his wife, he was badly stooped and his breathing was labored. He walked with a shuffle with his head pitched forward. His clenched fingers curled into his swollen hands. Norman guessed that he suffered from rheumatoid arthritis.

This day began as did other days. He went to the piano before going to the breakfast table. With difficulty he arranged himself on the piano bench. With noticeable effort he raised his swollen clenched fingers above the keyboard. His fingers slowly unlocked and reached toward the keys "like the buds of a plant toward the sunlight." His back straightened and he seemed to breathe more freely. He played some Bach with great sensitivity and control. Then he plunged into a Brahms concerto. His fingers were now agile and powerful as they raced across the keyboard with dazzling speed. His entire body seemed fused with the music. His body "was no longer stiff and shrunken but supple and graceful and completely freed of its arthritic coils." After the piece he stood up straighter and taller than before. He walked to the breakfast table without the shuffle, "ate heartily, talked animatedly, finished the meal, then went for a walk on the beach." Later the same day the same miracle occurred when he played his cello.

Norman added that Pablo Casals had "purpose, the will to live, faith, and good humor" which, adding to his creativity and his love for music from such composers as Bach, Brahms, Schubert, and Mozart, were important resources that enabled him to cope with his infirmities. Pablo Casals performed as a cellist and conductor well into his nineties.[28]

* * *

As humans we need to feel we have a genuine connectedness with others. We need to feel that there are people in our lives who care. Especially when our resources are low, feeling that someone cares can be essential to our very survival.

* * *

Jay Neugeboren interviewed people who recovered full lives after having been patients in psychiatric institutions for periods of ten or more years. These former patients included doctors, lawyers, teachers, social workers, and custodians. He asked them what had made the difference in their getting better. Whatever else they named, such as medications, finding God, a particular program, all said that a key element that brought them back was a relationship with a human being who in effect said, "I believe in your ability to recover, and I am going to stay with you until you do."[29]

* * *

A patient with last stage AIDS resisted all efforts to interact. A night nurse and an aide would not give up. They persisted in approaching him. He returned later looking healthy and said, "I started taking my meds again because someone was nice to me, and I realize I matter."[30]

* * *

Many of the stories have shown that getting the story right may mean including information from others who are there. If genuine interest is shown, it also tells them that they matter. How one gets that information is important. In Chapter 2, *Tell Me Your Story*, Debbie, the nurse on the airplane to California, on request from the flight attendant, talked with Arthur who had holed himself up in the bathroom. She said, "I really want to try and help you . . . . Could you come out, and we can sit down and talk?" You may remember that she and he did get a relationship whereby he came out, then slept through the rest of the trip when he lay down across the seats.

It is an abandonment of sorts to have one's thoughts and feelings ignored when they should reasonably be considered. The following story highlights this issue.

* * *

A linguistic researcher at a well known Northeastern hospital attended daily rounds for new doctors. At this rounds the attending physician proudly displayed to his audience all the lost skills of an elderly man who had recently suffered a stroke. "Look at how he cannot repeat after me, how he has trouble holding up two fingers, now three fingers . . . ." Then the doctor filled a small cup with water. He asked the patient to slowly raise it and drink from it. As he requested this action from the patient, he kept winking at the audience as if to say that the patient would not be able to respond to the request. The patient got the cup halfway to his mouth, then tossed the water all over the physician.[31]

* * *

Teachers are role models. How they handle their classes has a huge effect on their students, and whether or not the students feel they matter. This story about this teacher speaks for itself.

* * *

In her third grade math class, Deborah Ball started the day by calling on Sean. He said, "I was just thinking about six. I'm just thinking, it can be an odd number, too." Ball didn't shake her head. She just listened. Sean continued, speaking faster, "Cause there could be two, four, six, and two-three twos, that'd make six!" "Uh-huh," responded Ball. "And two threes," Sean added, now gaining steam. "It could be an odd and an even number. Both!" He looked up at his teacher in her black and red jumper and oversized glasses. She was sitting in a chair among her students. She continued to let him go on, never contradicting him. When he seemed to have stopped, she looked at the class. "Other people's comments?" she calmly asked.[32]

* * *

This teacher makes listening look easy. Sean is not concerned that his teacher will call him on being wrong, or being uncertain, or ignoring what doesn't fit. There is no hint of premature closure because he is supported for sorting through his thoughts, whatever they may be. His teacher encourages creative thinking in an environment that supports free flowing communication. We know that outside this classroom are environments not so supportive of his thinking. But this classroom environment can help him gain some sense of self and some resilience that can support him elsewhere.

Assumptions are shortcuts for our thinking and our behavior. We learn them early. We rely on them. It's difficult to recognize assumptions when assumptions are what we take for granted and accept as fact. But we need to try to recognize them if we want to be sure to get the story right, to be sure that we are on the same wavelength as the other person, to be sure that we truly understand the situation. If we don't recognize when we are making assumptions, we can at least make an effort to verify our thoughts and/or our feelings, to ascertain whether or not they make sense for the situation. Checklists can be helpful in routine situations, but even then the people involved need to contribute to them to own them and to communicate, as needed, to have them be useful.

To get the story right, the stories also tell us that too often we do not include information from the people that are there. Whose needs, ours or theirs? Maybe we both have needs. At least we need to try to recognize what is occurring with whatever information is available. We also need to understand each other to know that we matter to someone else and that we matter to ourselves.

The Orlando Communication Model tells us to first note our *Perceptions*, what we see, hear, taste, touch, or smell. Our problem is that we can quickly flow into our *Thoughts* and/or *Feelings* leaving us with our own interpretations that we may too quickly and decisively believe, then act upon. The next ingredient in her Model is *Validation*, so we can verify whether or not our interpretation is or is not correct. Then, if we follow through with an *Action,* we should again *Validate*, to be sure that our action has been correct for the situation.

If we make the effort to recognize our assumptions, or at least remember to *Verify*, the Orlando Model can help us get the story right.

21. One Final Story

As mentioned in Chapter 2, *Tell Me Your Story*, my grandfathers and my father were physicians before modern technology became available. They knew they had to communicate well with their patients and families to get the story right. Their offices were in their houses. Their house phones were their office phones. Most weeks they made house calls which contributed to knowing the life situations of their patients and their families. They gave much free care and were sometimes paid in local produce. I remember my father occasionally receiving venison during hunting season, a rare delicacy for our family.

My paternal grandfather, Victor Hugo Dye, M.D., practiced in Sistersville, West Virginia, a small town in oil drilling and coal mining country on the Ohio River. He not only made house calls in the hills of the area, he often took the ferry to see some of his hillbilly patients across the river. Over forty years after his death my husband and I visited Sistersville. When we took the ferry across to the Ohio shore, the ferryman easily acknowledged that he had heard about the well known, well liked Doc Dye. As we were leaving the Wells Inn on our last day, an elderly man was half limping, half running to the car while motioning for us not to leave. When he stopped to catch his breath, his first words were directed to me, "Are you Doc Dye's granddaughter?" He was delighted to have me ensure him that, yes, what he had heard was true, I am Doc Dye's granddaughter. He wanted me to know that he had known Doc Dye.

My maternal grandfather, Fred Ellsworth Clow, M.D., was in the last Harvard Medical School class that was admitted from high school directly into the medical school. Fred Clow practiced in Wolfeboro, New Hampshire, at first as a horse and buggy doctor. My mother remembered riding with him in a sleigh pulled by their horse on a cold, snowy winter day. My grandmother had warmed a brick from the coals of their wood stove, wrapped it in flannel, and put it at their feet to keep them warm. At a house call in the next town my mother held the ether cone for anesthesia when her father removed inflamed tonsils of a child who lay on the kitchen table. He preferred operating at the local hospital which he cofounded in 1907 when Teddy Roosevelt was President. But circumstances did not always allow him or his patients to get to the hospital. When I returned some forty years after his death, a local resident made a special effort to be sure I received my grandfather's office doorbell which is memorable for the huge indentation where his patients had pushed the push button on the bell so many times over and over again for so many years. It had come into possession of one of his relatives who had died who had not been able to part with it.

Fred Clow's hobby was collecting memorabilia on Abraham Lincoln. He slept in a replica of Lincoln's bed. Pictures of Lincoln, Lincoln's family, and others in that era covered his bedroom walls. He accepted many invitations to talk about Lincoln. His Lincoln Collection is now at Hildene, The Lincoln Family Home in Manchester, Vermont, the former mansion of Robert Todd Lincoln, Abe's eldest son. His astounding collection of artifacts includes hundreds of books, pictures, original newspaper articles and letters, and has filled a void for the Hildene collections. The Fred Ellsworth Clow's Collection can be found in Hildene's library with Robert Todd Lincoln's Collection.

My father, W. J. Paul Dye, M.D., F.A.C.S. (Fellow of the American College of Surgeons), was another Harvard Medical School graduate. He chose a number of residencies which resulted in his being qualified for a combined surgical, obstetric, and medical practice. During World War II he was the only surgeon in town with only one other physician who saw medical problems. Since the hospital did not have a staffed emergency service, he was often called for emergencies, though many people just came to the house and rang the office bell. The phone seemed to ring constantly. He supervised interns from Tufts Medical School in the late 1930s into the 1940s. Known as a gifted diagnostician and surgeon, I often heard of lives he saved, deliveries he made, and families who revered him. Though it is now over fifty years since his death, people still tell me they remember him from being his patients when they were children, or they will volunteer that "he delivered me . . . he was our family doctor," or, similar to the Sistersville comment, with surprise they'll want verification for: "Is it true that you're Doctor Dye's daughter?" When I first returned to work as a clinician in the county mental health clinic, some of my patients and families were related to those who were in my father's care. I'm not sure which one of us liked it more.

Though it would be reasonable to tell a story from any of these dedicated doctors, this quintessential story comes from the lore of my maternal grandfather, Dr. Fred Clow.

* * *

Elijah, Ephram, and Lettie ran the family farm with the help of Barnaby, their mixed Border Collie. The farm had been in the family for a few generations and had been handed down to Elijah and Ephram who were brothers. Lettie was Ephram's wife. Elijah had never married. They had a few cows from which they obtained their milk, selling the rest to neighbors. A couple dozen chickens roamed about from which they obtained eggs. Their rooster's early calls bothered no one, because they were used to getting up early. Their fields produced radishes, carrots, tomatoes, varieties of lettuce, and corn in season. In the fall their few apple trees produced a variety of delicious apples. The eggs and produce from the fields were sold at their farm stand as they were available.

The farm was in the foothills of the White Mountains and was surrounded by forest. They had some four acres, mostly tilled. Two draft horses helped till the fields and did other heavy pulling chores. Both Elijah and Ephram took care of the fields and drove the horses. Barnaby was useful herding the cows when they were in the pasture and were to come to the barn. Lettie took care of the chickens and collected the eggs. She managed their house, and you could usually find her in the kitchen. Her cooking was legendary. "Lettie's Apple Pies" in the fall were a specialty at the farm stand, and would be sold as soon as they were available.

Dr. Clow had known them for a number of years. He saw them on house visits for one ailment or another. They weren't ones to leave the farm unless they had to come into town. They lived some miles away from him, but he was efficient in his house calls by making other calls in their vicinity when he saw them. He had a car by now, and he enjoyed the ride through the woods and open fields.

Lately he'd been visiting Lettie. She had pneumonia which was doggedly lingering. He wanted to be sure she was on the mend. But it was Elijah that worried Ephram, not Lettie. For the past few years Ephram had told Dr. Clow that Elijah kept mumbling about some elves. Dr. Clow already knew Elijah saw some elves. Elijah had taken him to the barn to see the draft horses at his visit to Lettie when she first came down with the pneumonia. Elijah was usually taciturn, but in their brief conversation he said he saw some elves, but he didn't say they were bothering him. Ephram and Lettie knew Elijah saw them. Problem for Ephram was that no one else could see them.

When Dr. Clow had asked Elijah how much the elves bothered him, he had said, "Well, not enuff to do anythin . . . they don't bother me enuff to get in the way of my chores." So Dr. Clow tended to believe that even though Elijah occasionally mumbled about the elves, maybe they bothered Ephram more than they bothered Elijah. Even so, Dr. Clow often thought about Elijah and his elves, and he began to consider how to help him if he ever said the elves bothered him enough to get in the way of his chores.

Sure enough on this visit when he and Elijah were alone in the barn, Elijah said, "Doc, the elves have been botherin me. They've been gettin in the way of some of my chores." Dr. Clow told him that he'd been thinking about the elves. He looked down at Elijah, who was still looking up at him. "Elijah, suppose your elves might like to go to Boston?" Elijah looked down, then looked at his beloved draft horses and said, "Oh, I dunno, I dunno." He was briefly silent, then looked up at his doctor and with a serious expression said, "Well, I'll ask em."

Dr. Clow returned to the farm house and visited with Ephram who had seen his car and had come in from the fields. He was eating a piece of Lettie's famous apple pie, and was about ready to go when Elijah came in and said he'd like to talk with him before he left. "Okay, Elijah, be right with you." On their way to the car Elijah said, "The elves agreed, they'd like to go to Boston." "Okay, I'll arrange it. They can take the Sanbornville train. I'll be in touch." "Okay," said Elijah as his doctor climbed into his car.

A few days later Dr.Clow was on the phone. "It's all set, Elijah, I'll pick you and your elves up and we'll get them on the train to Boston." "Okay, Doc, we'll be waitin." Dr. Clow had been to the station and let the conductor know what he planned to do. At the appointed day and time Dr. Clow arrived at the farm and found

Elijah standing outside in clean coveralls, his favorite red flannel shirt, and the navy crushed hat he always wore. Elijah opened the back door of the car and let the elves into the back seat. Elijah got in front and they all headed toward Sanbornville. The ride was quiet until they were almost there. Then all of a sudden Elijah said: "Doc Clow, what about the tickets!" "All arranged, Elijah, the conductor has them."

They met the conductor at the station. Elijah opened the car's back door and waited until the elves were out, then closed the door. Elijah and the elves went over to the train. Elijah nodded to the conductor who was standing on the landing by the train door. The elves boarded the train. The conductor followed. The train whistled and slowly started to move. Elijah and Doc Clow watched the train gain steam, strain around the first bend, then disappear out of sight as it whistled and rolled on to Boston.

Some time later Dr. Clow returned to the farm to be sure Lettie no longer had her pneumonia, also to see how things were going. Elijah took their doctor back to the barn, his favorite place to visit with him. He was his usual taciturn self, but finally looked up and with a grin and slight nod said, "Doc Clow. I been wantin to tell ya. Haven't seen the elves since the train. They must like Boston." Dr. Clow looked down at Elijah and responded with his own grin. He nodded and softly said, "That's good, Elijah. That's good."

* * *

Appendix A
Relaxation-Meditation Exercise: Talking to Your T-Cells[1]
(T-cells from the thymus gland are important fighters in the body's immune response to foreign cells.)

This relaxation-meditation exercise can be done with or without music. If you choose music, consider Pachelbel's Canon in D Major for strings. The music should be peaceful and relaxing for you. It should be at a low volume so it will not overcome your thoughts. Most people ultimately choose a quiet setting without music.

* * *

Get in a comfortable chair (such as a lounge chair) with your legs, knees, and feet raised (by the lounge chair or supported by a stool). Your knees should be flexed in a comfortable position. Your arms and hands should be at ease in your lap.

Close your eyes. Take a deep breath to help you relax. Slowly and deeply breathe in and out at least five times, counting (quietly to yourself) one thousand in, one thousand out, two thousand in, two thousand out, and the like through five thousand. Do this however long you need until you feel relaxed. It is important that you feel comfortable enough not to change your position throughout the exercise.

Focus on your toes and tell them to tingle. If they do not, focus on your fingers and tell them to tingle. (If you feel your toes or fingers tingle, you have proof that your body responds to your thoughts. Whether or not this occurs continue with the exercise.)

Now visualize a peaceful place where you like to be. It could be by a lake, ocean, or some other place. Pick your own special place. Whatever you choose, continue to visualize it and, as in a picture, fill in the details about that place. As you visualize yourself there, see the sun streaming down and warming you all over. See yourself relaxed and comfortable there.

Now focus on the thymus gland (it resembles a walnut, so imagine it) in the lower part of your neck just behind the upper part of the breastbone. Visualize your T-cells as tiny round tennis balls in the thymus gland changing into active T-cells like an aloe plant with succulent leaves all around it. Visualize these active T-cells going through your body to any specific place you know that has any abnormal cells. Visualize them nibbling on and destroying any of these foreign cells at those specific places. (The Pac Man, somewhat like a V opening and closing, is a favorite image, or choose a mental picture you like.)

Continue to visualize your T-cells destroying the foreign cells. With your same image, tell them to go anywhere in your body and destroy any other foreign cells. Give them time to do this. Just before you finish this exercise, tell them to continue to do their work.

When you are ready, or when the music is finished, you can open your eyes and begin to awaken your body by stretching your arms and legs. At your own pace, you can decide when to stand up and move on with your day.

* * *

The exercise should be done a minimum of ten minutes once a day. Because our bodies like habit try to choose the same time each day. Your body will get used to your doing it then. This is biofeedback which you can use to assist any healing process, such as with fractures, infections, and viruses. Visualize that part of your body healing with whatever images make sense for the situation. Also, tell your body to continue with the healing as you go on with your day.

Even when you are not doing this relaxation-meditation exercise, you can take a few deep breaths and visualize your special place. During such time you can talk to your T-cells to support their working for you. Also, in your mind you can quietly play relaxing music. If you turn to the same music to help you relax, your body will come to know it as a signal to relax. Since it is impossible to think more than one thing at a time, if you want to slow down, or move out unwanted thoughts or feelings, play your own comforting music in your head. Unless you choose to tell someone that you do this, no one but you will know.

Remember that our bodies like habit. The more consistently you do any of this, the easier it is to do. Since the mind's influence on our health is well documented in the research from psychoneuroimmunology, meditation and relaxation techniques can assist us in supporting good health and in dealing with stresses in our lives.

Appendix B
Conversations with Orlando and the Author

Innumerable conversations with Ida Orlando over the years until her death in 2007 prompt me to share some of her thoughts about her theory, clarifications that she was aware were needed.

Some people believed Orlando was influenced by other thinkers. She emphatically denied this. She wanted people to know that she went to the hospital and observed nurse-patient interactions without any preconceived ideas. She believed such observations were essential data to help her figure out what differentiated "good nursing" that responded to and met patients' needs from "bad nursing" that did not meet patients' needs (see Chapter 3, *Orlando's Enigma*). Orlando realized that good communication is a process. She discovered the ingredients (*Perceptions*, *Thoughts*, *Feelings*, *Validation*, *Action*) in the "good nursing". These are discussed in full in Chapter 19, *Recognizing Assumptions*.

She would sometimes refer to the good communication that she discovered in the interactions as The Process. She did not want her students to refer to The Process as Orlando's Process because that was not accurate. She would say, "It's their process, not mine. It's what they think in the situation, not what I think." She emphasized that they needed to capture their own thoughts and feelings and check out the validity of any thoughts, feelings, or actions that they took in the situation. "They were there, I wasn't there," she'd say.

When I told her that some students of The Process were asking for "tools", she and I both knew that they misunderstood The Process. In analyzing situations with her students she would ask them to remember and discuss what they were thinking and feeling in the situation as it evolved. She would remind them that "Situations are unique. People can attend to what is happening and be aware of their own thoughts and feelings. Those are their tools." She realized "It takes discipline to attend to what is going on, and the ability to attend to what is occurring improves the more you make the effort to stay in the moment and focus on what is happening." In other words, it becomes easier to do the more you do it.

Many have asked why her Model seems so difficult to practice when it appears so simple. This book discusses this in great detail, most especially in Chapter 20, *Reflections*. Orlando realized that recognizing assumptions was a core issue. Also, we can too easily behave mindlessly rather than mindfully. Sherlock Holmes said to Dr. Watson, "I have trained myself to notice what I see."[1] We could do well to do the same, which means that throughout The Process it is important to note our *Perceptions*, the raw data in front of us, the data that we are aware of through any of our senses: what we see, hear, taste, touch, or smell. Once we interpret this data we have moved to our *Thoughts* and/or *Feelings*. Until we *Validate*, or verify, those thoughts or feelings for accuracy, they are only our unique interpretations. The stories in this book show what happens when we make and act on incorrect assumptions. We just don't get the story right.

Orlando and I never discussed how early one might begin to help children in getting the story right. Chapter 9, *The Need to be Heard* includes stories relevant to this issue. Getting the story right begins with good parenting, regardless of who is in the role of caretaker. Good role models who get the story right will help children learn how to get the story right. They can learn what it means to verify, to support what they are saying with reasonable information. For example, "Did your teacher really say that, or is that what you think she meant? You're not sure? Then let's talk about your going back and asking your teacher what was meant."

KIPP (Knowledge Is Power Program) began with fifth graders. In class the students learn the rubric of SLANT (Sit up straight, Look and Listen, Ask and Answer questions, Nod your head if you understand, and Track the speaker). Slogans posted on the walls of KIPP schools include "Work hard. Be nice."[2] Such programs which include verification can assist children in getting the story right. Their basics support good communication which includes accurate understanding of what is occurring.

Orlando and I never discussed multi-tasking. However, it is important to know that continually responding to Internet distractions affects attention and the ability to focus. It changes our brain patterns, our brain pathways. Nicholas Carr in *The Shallows: What the Internet is Doing to Our Brains* is worth reading in this regard. He states the following. "Dozens of people wrote to share . . . how the Web has scattered their attention, parched their memory, or turned them into compulsive nibblers of info-snacks."

He mentions that a large number of those in high school, college, and in their twenties have told him they fear that the "constant connectivity may be constricting rather than expanding their horizons." A college senior sent him a long e-mail which described how he has struggled "with a moderate to major form of Internet addiction since the third grade." This college senior said that he is drawn back into the Web even though he knows that "the happiest and most fulfilled times of my life have all involved a prolonged separation from the Internet."[3]

Nicholas Carr also discussed how, when he began writing *The Shallows*, he could not stay focused on the task. The Net's "constant interruptions scattered my thoughts and words. I tended to write in disconnected spurts, the same way I wrote when blogging." He continued to say that "for months my synapses howled for their next fix." He persevered in staying away from the Web and "in time the cravings subsided." He added "Some old, disused neural circuits were springing back to life . . . . I started to feel generally calmer and more in control of my thoughts . . . . My brain could breathe again."[4]

We have long known that, for ourselves physically: if we don't use it we lose it. We might also keep in mind that now we know that there is evidence that says the same for our brain, the more often we make an effort to stay in the moment, focus and verify as needed, we progressively will find it easier to get the story right.

Appendix C
Robert J. and Ida Orlando Pelletier Memorial Service

On September 7, 2012, colleagues, friends, and family attended the Robert J. and Ida Orlando Pelletier Memorial Service at the Bigelow Chapel, Mount Auburn Cemetery, Cambridge, Massachusetts. Prior to the Service, family and invited guests attended the burial of their ashes at the Cemetery.

During the Service, mostly through stories, various friends and colleagues of Bob and Ida shared their memories. The Yale University School of Nursing invited me to attend the Service on their behalf. As if I were talking with Ida, the following is what I shared.

* * *

Ida, about ten days ago I accepted an invitation from the Yale University School of Nursing to be their delegate at this Service to honor you. They may know I was a student of yours in two of the master degree programs. But they may not know about the close friendship we developed over the years. A praiseworthy obituary about you was in their Spring 2008 Alunmae/i Magazine. Included were three marvelous pictures of you when you were young, just as I remember you when you were teaching our classes. When you first came into our seminar room you blew me away with your enormous energy and charisma. You were passionate about good patient care. You wrote on the blackboard in large block letters: Never Assume.

As you know, those were the years when you worked on your manuscript that resulted in your first book. We loved your telling us that you put the manuscript in your refrigerator when you weren't working on it. You said you did not want it destroyed if your apartment got on fire.

By the mid-nineties you and I began to have long conversations. I was on the Rivier College faculty and told you about a required graduate nursing course that included all the nursing theories. Some of the students asked me to participate in an Orlando Theory Video for their class project. They knew I had been a student of yours. They wanted me to answer their questions about Orlando Theory. They also admitted that the students in the class believed that Orlando Theory was more relevant for their practice than any of the other nursing theories.

I told them to give me their questions, and I'd ask you if you would answer them. Oh, they loved that idea. You said of course you would. And so you did. In the video they asked more questions than they had listed for you. I made it clear which of the answers were yours and which ones were mine. It wasn't surprising that they received an A+ for their project. Later I sent the video to you, and you laughed when I said you had been as disciplined in your observations as had Jane Goodall with the chimpanzees and Dian Fossey with the gorillas.

For about a decade which began in the late nineties you know that I was a consultant on Orlando Theory at New Hampshire Hospital, the acute psychiatric hospital in Concord, New Hampshire. Your theory had been voted on by the nursing and mental health staff as being more relevant for their practice than any of the other nursing theories they reviewed. Sounds similar to what the Rivier students said, doesn't it? The staff put into practice your theory which has resulted in less use of seclusion rooms and less acting out by patients. The staff and patients are now more satisfied with the care, and some of the doctors have shown keen interest in why this has occurred.

At New Hampshire Hospital I gave a speech about Orlando Theory to a large staff group. One person demanded to know why schools of nursing, medicine, and business don't know about this. Another person came to the speech to learn more. She said it was valuable in her personal life.

Then, in March 2007 I told you that the Wellesley College Club on the Wellesley College Campus asked me to give a lecture at the Club in an evening lecture series. I am an alum, but I didn't know what they wanted me to talk about. They said they didn't care. So, using various stories as illustrations, I told them what Orlando Theory can offer us, all of us, where ever we are, whatever we are doing. Various people stopped and talked with me after the lecture. Two doctors believed Orlando Theory could improve medical practice. Some lay people told me they believed they would communicate better if they were aware of their assumptions, and they continued to mumble about that as they went out the door. Three student teachers said they were fascinated by my lecture, and added that they planned to use Orlando Theory the next morning in their student teaching.

That lecture was in March 2008. You and Bob had planned to be there. But by then you had moved on. Bob came with two of your nursing friends. We really missed you on that successful evening when it was obvious that Orlando Theory was embraced by doctors as well as others who were not in health care.

Later Bob told me that a participant at one of your conferences in Canada had struggled with a situation. So, with much emphasis, another participant had said: "Just do an Orlando." I am aware that more and more health systems are teaching their staff to "Just do an Orlando." Also, I am aware that many of those who know Orlando Theory are using it in their lives.

Bob chuckled when he told me someone had called him Mr. Orlando, and that he welcomed being an Orlando husband. Because my husband now knows Orlando Theory from me, he recognizes assumptions and prides himself on being my Orlando husband.

I believe that the Yale University School of Nursing is aware that your legacy is growing. I was blessed to be a student of yours so many years ago, then a colleague, and close friend.

All for now Ida. But, now and again, you know I will share my thoughts with you.

Notes and References

References have been consolidated to reduce the number of citations. Pages cited include quotes, specific information in the text, and/or information relevant to the topic under consideration. After a citation is listed in full, if it reoccurs it is listed only in brief. Most reference numbers are at the end of the relevant texts.

I was a student, then colleague and close friend of Ida Orlando until her death in 2007. She encouraged and supported me in writing this book because she acknowledged that I not only understood her theory, I knew the content of her books and the difficulties in putting her theory into practice. She said, "You know my theory as well as I do, go ahead and do what you want with it." Therefore, since my understanding about her theory inevitably comes mostly from our innumerable conversations over the years, Reference #2 in the Preface is the only Orlando reference.

Preface

1. Institute of Medicine (IOM). (2000). *To Err is Human: Building a Safer Health System*. Washington, DC: National Academy Press. especially pp. 1-5, 26-48.
2. Orlando, I.J. (1961). *The Dynamic Nurse-Patient Relationship*. New York, NY: G.P. Putnam's Sons. [Reissued in 1990. New York, NY: National League for Nursing.] [Original Project at the Yale University School of Nursing, New Haven, CT.] / Orlando, I.J. (1972). *The Discipline and Teaching of Nursing Process*. New York, NY: G.P. Putnam's Sons. [An Evaluative Study at McLean Hospital, Belmont, MA.]
3. Yale University School of Medicine Alumnae College. (06-04-1983). This author's notes from a lecture and slide presentation where psychoneuroimmunology (PNI) was the focus. The slides included pictures of inactive and active T-cells. Studies presented showed the mind's influence on T-cell function. In one such study people in one group who told their T-cells to go to a specific cancer location had more T-cells there and more often had a remission of their cancer as compared to those in another group that did not do this. / Locke, S. & D. Colligan. (1986). *The Healer Within: The New Medicine of Mind and Body*. New York, NY: E.P. Dutton. pp. 27-59. / Siegel, B.S. (1986). *Love, Medicine & Miracles*. New York, NY: Harper & Row. pp. 147-156. / Siegel, B.S. (1989). *Peace, Love & Healing*. New York, NY: Harper & Row. pp. 109-115. / Simonton, O.C., S. Matthews-Simonton & J.L. Creighton. (1978). *Getting Well Again*. New York, NY: Bantam Books. pp. 6-8, 119-126.

1. Orlando's Model

1. Warsh, D. (09-17-1995). Molecular Medicine vs. Bedside Manner in the Lehman Case. *The Boston Sunday Globe*. pp. 79, 83. / Gorman, C. (04-03-1995). The Disturbing Case of the Cure That Killed the Patient. *Time*. pp. 60-61. / Knox, R.A. (07-16-1995). Hospital's Record of Sympathy Faulted. *The Boston Sunday Globe*. pp. 21, 27.

2. Tell Me Your Story

1. Dobkin, B. (10-1990). The Sit-In. *Discover*. pp. 22, 28.
2. Smith, D.J. (10-2000). Flight to Los Angeles. *Journal of Psychosocial Nursing*. vol. 38, no. 10. pp. 38-43.

4. Urgent!

1. Thomas, E. (04-30-2007). Making of a Massacre. *Newsweek.* pp. 22-31. / Guardian Reporters. (04-20 to 26, 2007). Campus Shooting the Deadliest in US History. *The Guardian Weekly.* vol. 176, no. 18. p. 1.
2. New York Times Reporter. (07-15-2007). State Dispatchers Dismissed Early 911 Reports of Tahoe Fire. *National: The New York Times.* p. 17.

6. Automatic Assumptions Can Mislead

1. CNN. (10-12-2009).Television News. / NECN. (10-13-2009). Television News. Headline at Bottom of Screen.
2. ABC. (04-14-2009). Television News. / CNN & NECN. (04-15-2009). Television News. / Belluck, P. (04-26-2009). Yes, Looks Do Matter. *Sunday Styles: The New York Times.* pp. 1, 8. / Newsweek Reporter. (04-27-2009). *Viral Video: Newsweek.* p. 19. / Heffernan, V. (06-28-09). The Susan Boyle Experience. *The New York Times Magazine.* pp. 16, 18.

7. Betrayed

1. Greland-Goldstein, J. (09-2009). Way Station. *American Journal of Nursing.* vol. 109, no. 9. p. 80.

8. Now Will You Listen

1. CNN & ABC. (11-28-2007). Television News. [These stations periodically followed the events for some 5 hours until the situation was resolved.] / ABC. (12-02-2007; 12-03-2007; 12-05-2007; 12-06-2007). Television News. / Viser, M. & J. Pindell. (12-02-2007). Troubled Picture of N.H. Man Emerges. *City & Region: The Boston Sunday Globe.* pp. B 1, B 7.

10. Acknowledge Me

1. Jones, C.P. (03-1994). In Sam's Shop. *American Journal of Nursing.* pp. 50-52.
2. Miller, S. (04-2004). Making A Connection. *Clinician News.* p. 14.

11. Respect Me

1. Wright, L. (06-14-2004). Spending Summers with 'Super Grampy'. *My Turn: Newsweek.* p. 18.
2. Scotty, C. (10-18-2004). Can I Get You Some Manners With That? *My Turn: Newsweek.* p. 24.
3. Rogers, T. (12-11-2000). Fellow Nerds: Let's Celebrate Nerdiness! *My Turn: Newsweek.* p. 14.

12. Our Doctors Need Our Stories

1. Sanders, L. (2009). *Every Patient Tells A Story.* New York, NY: Broadway Books. pp. xxvi, 6.
2. Osler, W. (Third Edition 02-1932. Reprinted 03-1953.) *Aequanimitas.* New York, NY: The Blakiston Co. p. 315. [First Edition 10-06-1904.]
3. Groopman, J. (2007). *How Doctors Think.* New York, NY: Houghton Mifflin Co. pp. 59-63.
4. Groopman, J. *How Doctors Think.* p. 67.
5. Groopman, J. *How Doctors Think.* pp. 3, 47-48.
6. Nuland, S.B. (2010). The Internist's Tale. *The Soul of Medicine.* New York, NY: Kaplan. pp. 147-154.
7. IOM. *To Err Is Human.* pp. xi, 1.
8. Sanders, L. *Every Patient Tells A Story.* pp. 215, xxii.
9. Groopman, J. *How Doctors Think.* p. 24.
10. Sanders, L. *Every Patient Tells A Story.* p. 230.
11. Sanders, L. *Every Patient Tells A Story.* p. xxiv. / Groopman, J. *How Doctors Think.* pp. 171, 260, 263.

13. How We Hear Our Doctors

1. Nuland, S.B. The Pediatrician's Tale. *The Soul of Medicine*. pp. 193-196.
2. Lown, B. (1999). *The Lost Art of Healing*. New York, NY: Ballantine Books. pp. 61-63.
3. Lown, B. *The Lost Art of Healing*. pp. 81-82.
4. Siegel, B.S. *Peace, Love & Healing*. pp. 86-87.
5. Rossi, E.L. (1993). *The Psychobiology of Mind-Body Healing*. New York, NY: W.W. Norton & Co. pp. 4-6.
6. Lown, B. *The Lost Art of Healing*. pp. 83-85.
7. Nuland, S.B. The Cardiologist's Tale. *The Soul of Medicine*. pp. 55-63.
8. Same references as those listed for Reference #3 in Preface.

14. When We Are Patients

1. Gallin, P.F. (2003). *How To Survive Your Doctor's Care*. Washington, DC: LifeLine Press. pp. xiii-xvi.
2. Groopman, J. (2000). *Second Opinions*. New York, NY: Penguin Books. pp. 36-37.
3. Groopman, J. *Second Opinions*. pp. 1-4.
4. Gawande, A. (2002). *Complications*. New York, NY: Henry Holt and Co. pp. 224-227.
5. Butler, K. (06-20-2010). My Father's Broken Heart. *The New York Times Magazine*. pp. 38-43.
6. Sanders, L. *Every Patient Tells A Story*. pp. 41-42, 75-76.
7. Katz, J. (1984 with new material 2002). *The Silent World of Doctor and Patient*. Baltimore, MD: The Johns Hopkins University Press. especially pp. xxxvii, 112, xix.
8. Schneider, C.E. (1998). *The Practice of Autonomy: Patients, Doctors, and Medical Decisions*. New York, NY: Oxford University Press. especially pp. 195, 181.

15. Hospitals

1. Kirkland, L.R. (06-2007). 'Them' and 'Us': A View from the Middle. *American Journal of Nursing*. vol. 107, no. 6. pp. 58-59.
2. Groopman, J. *How Doctors Think*. pp. 54-56.
3. Cousins, N. (05/06-1983). Why is Norman Cousins Smiling . . . Again? *American Health*. pp. 56-64.
4. Payne, D. (08-22-2005). I Shouldn't Have Had To Beg for a Prognosis. *My Turn: Newsweek*. p. 16.

16. Hospitals and Hierarchies

1. IOM. *To Err Is Human*. pp. 1, 6, 49, 52-53, 65, 180.
2. Beck, C.T. (04-1998). Intuition in Nursing Practice: Sharing Graduate Students' Exemplars With Undergraduate Students. *Journal of Nursing Education*. vol. 37, no. 4. pp. 169-172. especially p. 171.
3. Pronovost, P. & E. Vohr. (2010). *Safe Patients, Smart Hospitals*. New York, NY: Penguin Group. pp. 73-77.
4. Salamon, J. (2008). *Hospital*. New York, NY: The Penguin Press. pp. 220-241. Story pp. 230-231.
5. Karl, R.C. (09-24-2007). Good Doctors Spot Mistakes, Save Lives. *My Turn: Newsweek*. p. 24.
6. Pronovost, P. & E. Vohr. *Safe Patients, Smart Hospitals*. p. 83.
7. Pronovost, P. & E. Vohr. *Safe Patients, Smart Hospitals*. especially pp. 17-30, 48-51, 94-97.
8. Pronovost, P. & E. Vohr. *Safe Patients, Smart Hospitals*. p. 135.
9. Pronovost, P. & E. Vohr. *Safe Patients, Smart Hospitals*. p. 224.

10. Hallinan, J.T. (2009). *Why We Make Mistakes*. New York, NY: Broadway Books. p.194.
11. Hallinan, J.T. *Why We Make Mistakes*. p. 195.
12. Pronovost, P. & E. Vohr. *Safe Patients, Smart Hospitals*. p. 82.
13. Curtin, L. (07-2010). Going from the Gut. *American Nurse Today*. vol. 5, no. 7. p. 48.
14. Gawande, A. (2009). *The Checklist Manifesto*. New York, NY: Henry Holt and Co. pp. 86-173. especially pp. 88, 173, 159.
15. Pronovost, P. & E. Vohr. *Safe Patients, Smart Hospitals*. pp. 233-238. / Gawande, A. *The Checklist Manifesto*. pp. 140-141. / Salamon, J. *Hospital*. pp. 226-227.
16. Gawande, A. *The Checklist Manifesto*. pp. 108-109.
17. Salamon, J. *Hospital*. pp. 226-227.
18. Gawande, A. *The Checklist Manifesto*. p. 79.
19. Stotland, E. & A.L. Kobler. (1965). *Life and Death of a Mental Hospital*. Seattle, WA: University of Washington Press. p. 241.

17. Hierarchies

1. Uchitelle, L. (04-01-2007). The End of the Line as They Know It. *Sunday Business: The New York Times*. pp. 1, 9-10.
2. Alderman, L. (10-10-2010). A Shoemaker That Walks But Never Runs. *Sunday Business: The New York Times*. pp. 1, 7. / Nadeau, B.L. (07-25-2011). Italy's Luxury Bailout. *Newsweek*. pp. 52-58. [More information about Diego Della Valle and Tod's.]
3. Gladwell, M. (2000). *The Tipping Point*. New York, NY: Little, Brown and Co. pp. 182-192.
4. Wolf, M.L. (07-23-2006). A Death Foreshadowed? *Opinion: Boston Sunday Globe*. p. E 9.
5. Pereli, D. (07-23-2006). *Letters to the Editor: Boston Sunday Globe*. p. E 10.
6. Gawande, A. *The Checklist Manifesto*. pp. 54-71.
7. Estabrook, B. (10-10-2010). The Catch. *The New York Times Magazine*. pp. 44-47, 76, 78.

18. The Milieu in Health Care

1. Stoddard, S. (1978). *The Hospice Movement*. New York, NY: Vintage Books. / Sarton, M. (1988). *After the Stroke: A Journal*. New York, NY: W.W. Norton & Co. especially pp. 23-24, 42-43, 70, 73, 76-77, 104-107.
2. Nuland, S.B. The Neurologist's Tale(s). *The Soul of Medicine*. especially pp. 176-178.
3. Iyengar, S. (2010). *The Art of Choosing*. New York, NY: Twelve, Hachette Book Group. pp. 16-18.
4. Neushotz, L.A., L.V. Green & P.S. Matos. (09/10-2009). How Dolls Can Help Patients with Dementia. *American Nurse Today*. vol. 4, no. 8. pp. 36-37.
5. Nuland, S.B. (2003). *Lost in America*. New York, NY: Alfred A. Knopf. pp. 79-83.
6. Frampton, S.B. (03-2009). Creating a Patient-Centered System. *American Journal of Nursing*. vol. 109, no. 3. pp. 30-33.
7. The Hospice Information is from conversations with Florence Wald and the following: Stoddard, S. *The Hospice Movement*. especially pp. 165-169, 199, 218-225, 285. / Rossman, P. (1977). *Hospice*. New York, NY: Fawcett Columbine Books. especially pp. 118-127. /Obituary Information is from the following: In Memoriam, Ida Jean Orlando (1926-2007): *Yale Nursing Matters*. Spring 2008. vol. 8, no. 2. p. 27. In Memoriam, Florence S. Wald (1917-2008): *Yale Nursing Matters*. Spring 2009. vol. 9, no. 2. p. 18.
8. Sternberg, E.M. (2009). *Healing Spaces: The Science of Place and Well-Being*. Cambridge, MA.: The Belknap Press of Harvard University Press. especially

Chapter 10: Hospitals and Well-Being. pp. 215-252. Statement in text is from pp. 244-245.

19. Recognizing Assumptions

1. Nuland, S.B. The Neurologist's Tale(s). *The Soul of Medicine*. p. 175.
2. Spiro, H.M., M.G. McCrea Curnen, E. Peschel & D. St. James. (Editors). (1993). *Empathy and the Practice of Medicine*. New Haven, CT: Yale University Press. / Sanders, L. *Every Patient Tells A Story*. / Groopman, J. *How Doctors Think*. / Charon, R. (2006). *Narrative Medicine*. New York, NY: Oxford University Press.
3. Spiro, H.M., et al. *Empathy and the Practice of Medicine*. p. 4.
4. Sanders, L. *Every Patient Tells A Story*. p. 6
5. Groopman, J. *How Doctors Think*. pp. 7-8.
6. Charon, R. *Narrative Medicine*. p. vii.
7. Sanders, L. *Every Patient Tells A Story*. pp. 153-154.
8. Sanders, L. *Every Patient Tells A Story*. p. 154.
9. Sanders, L. *Every Patient Tells A Story*. pp. 92-94.
10. Kowalczyk, L. (07-20-2008). Monet? Gauguin? Using Art to Make Better Doctors. *Boston Sunday Globe*. pp. A 1, A 14.
11. Belluz, J. (11-15-2010). Out of the Hospital and into the Museum. *Mclean's Magazine*. pp. 56, 58.
12. McKie, R. (09-23-2011). The Artist Will See You Now. *The Guardian Weekly*. pp. 32-33.
13. Belluz, J. Out of the Hospital and into the Museum. pp. 56, 58.
14. Glick, S.M. The Empathic Physician: Nature and Nurture. Spiro, H.M., et al. *Empathy and the Practice of Medicine*. pp. 85-102. especially pp. 96-99. [Information re: S.M. Glick. pp. 194-195.]
15. Halpern, J. Empathy: Using Resonance Emotions in the Service of Curiosity. Spiro, H.M., et al. *Empathy and the Practice of Medicine*. pp. 160-173. especially p. 162. [Information re: J. Halpern. p. 195.]
16. Zagier, A.S. (03-14-2010). Book Clubs Show Human Side of Medicine. *Lifestyles: New Hampshire Sunday News*. p. F 9.
17. Powers, J. (Fall, 2009). Looking Is Not Seeing, Listening Is Not Hearing. *Yale Nursing Matters*. vol. 10, no. 1. pp. 11-13. especially pp. 11-12.
18. Hirschfeld, N. (10-2009). Teaching Cops to See. *Smithsonian*. pp. 48-54. especially pp. 49, 54.
19. Wallace, L. (01-10-2010). Multicultural Critical Theory. At B-School? *The New York Times*. pp. 1, 7.

20. Reflections

1. Olbrych, D.D.V. (12-2002). Inseparable. *American Journal of Nursing*. vol. 102, no. 12. p. 25.
2. Groopman, J. *Second Opinions*. pp. 9-34.
3. Groopman, J. *Second Opinions*. pp. 35-36.
4. Groopman, J. *How Doctors Think*. p. 10.
5. IOM. *To Err Is Human*. p. 174.
6. Sanders, L. *Every Patient Tells A Story*. Various pages to include pp. 7, 92, 198, 201-202, 207-208, 230. / Groopman, J. *How Doctors Think*. Various pages to include pp. 35, 44, 56-57, 65, 238-239, 263.
7. Katz, J. *The Silent World of Doctor and Patient*. p. 184.
8. Tannen, D. (1994). *Talking From 9 to 5*. New York, NY: William Morrow and Co. p. 26.
9. Tannen, D. *Talking From 9 to 5*. p. 26.
10. Tannen, D. *Talking From 9 to 5*. pp. 24-25.
11. Tannen, D. *Talking From 9 to 5*. pp. 28-29.
12. Gawande, A. (2007). *Better*. New York, NY: Henry Holt and Co. pp. 23-27.
13. Salamon, J. *Hospital*. p. 41.

14. Garber, K. (11-2009). Planting the Seeds for Advances on Energy. *U.S. News & World Report.* p. 69.
15. Bryant, A. (11-01-2009). Leadership Without a Secret Code. *Sunday Business: The New York Times.* p. 2.
16. Isenalumhe, A. E. (01-2000). Using Therapeutic Support: My Hands-On Experience as a Psychiatric Nurse. *Journal of Psychosocial Nursing.* vol. 38, no. 1. pp. 23-26. especially p. 24.
17. Sarton, M. *After the Stroke.* p. 101.
18. Maclean, N. (1992). *Young Men and Fire.* Chicago, IL: The University of Chicago Press. pp. 31-109. / Lehrer, J. (07-28-2008). The Eureka Hunt: Why Do Good Ideas Come To Us When They Do? *The New Yorker.* pp. 40-45.
19. Latner, A.W. (11-2008). A Patient's Belligerence Rattles PA. *The Clinical Advisor.* pp. 98-99.
20. Tavris, C. & E. Aronson. (2007). *Mistakes Were Made (but not by me).* New York, NY: Harcourt. p. 220.
21. Kalb, C. (10-16-2006). Fixing America's Hospitals: Facing Up To Mistakes. *Newsweek.* pp. 44, 46, 49.
22. IOM. *To Err Is Human.* p. 1. [Colorado and Utah Study: extrapolated to 44,000. New York Study: extrapolated to 98,000.]
23. Gawande, A. *Better.* p. 107.
24. Gladwell, M. (2005). *Blink.* New York, NY: Little, Brown and Co. p. 40.
25. Gladwell, M. *Blink.* pp. 41-43.
26. Lown, B. *The Lost Art of Healing.* p.149.
27. Tavris, C. & E. Aronson. *Mistakes Were Made (but not by me).* p. 219.
28. Cousins, N. (1979). *Anatomy of an Illness as Perceived by the Patient.* New York, NY: W.W. Norton & Co. pp. 79-88.
29. Neugeboren, J. (02-06-2006). Meds Alone Couldn't Bring Robert Back. *My Turn: Newsweek.* p. 17.
30. Keefe, S. (05-04-2009). Maintaining Their Dignity. *Advance for Nurses: New England.* pp. 22-23. especially p. 22.
31. Behrens, S.J. (05-15-2011). When Doctors Humiliate Nurses: To The Editor. *Sunday Opinion: The New York Times.* p. 7.
32. Green, E. (03-07-2010). Can Good Teaching Be Learned? *The New York Times Magazine.* pp. 30-37, 44, 46. especially pp. 36-37.

Appendix A
Relaxation-Meditation Exercise: Talking to Your T-Cells

1. Same references as those listed for Reference #3 in Preface.

Appendix B
Conversations with Orlando and the Author

1. Sanders, L. *Every Patient Tells A Story.* p. 90.
2. Mathews, J. (2009). *Work Hard. Be Nice.* Chapel Hill, NC: Algonquin Books of Chapel Hill. [This book discusses the KIPP Program: its origin, trials and tribulations with discussion and description of the model. SLANT is discussed on pp. 73, 153.] / Whitman, D. (2008). Kipp Academy. *Sweating the Small Stuff.* Washington, DC: Thomas B. Fordham Institute Press. pp. 150-189. [SLANT is discussed on p. 101.]
3. Carr, N. (2010). *The Shallows: What the Internet is Doing to Our Brains.* New York, NY: W.W. Norton & Co. p. 226.
4. Carr, N. *The Shallows.* especially pp. 180-197 regarding changes in the brain. especially pp. 198-200 where N. Carr discusses his struggles in writing this book.

The Author

Mary C. (Mimi) Dye has a B.A. degree from Wellesley College, an M.N. degree and an M.S.N. degree from the Yale University School of Nursing. Her career has included: Associate Professor and Chair of the Psychiatric Mental Health Nursing Program at the Yale University School of Nursing with a joint faculty appointment at the Connecticut Mental Health Center serving as clinician, clinical supervisor, and psychotherapist on inpatient, outpatient, and emergency services; Clinical Director of the Wolfeboro, New Hampshire, Office of the Northern New Hampshire Mental Health Center serving as administrator, supervisor, psychotherapist, and clinician in emergency services; member of a professional delegation to the People's Republic of China with the People to People Ambassador Program; Associate Professor, Rivier College, Nashua, New Hampshire; and consultant for the Nursing Department of New Hampshire Hospital, Concord, New Hampshire, implementing Orlando Theory into clinical practice. As an Advanced Practice Registered Nurse she has been, and continues to be, a consultant and psychotherapist in private practice. She resides with her husband, David Dunham, in Wolfeboro, New Hampshire.